COGNITIVE-BEHAVIORAL THERAPY
FOR IMPULSIVE CHILDREN

Cognitive-Behavioral Therapy for Impulsive Children

Second Edition

Philip C. Kendall
Lauren Braswell

THE GUILFORD PRESS
New York   London

Published by the Guilford Press
A Division of Guilford Publications, Inc.
72 Spring Street, New York, NY 10012

Printed in the United States of America

This book is printed on acid-free paper.

Last digit is print number: 9   8   7   6   5

Library of Congress Cataloging-in-Publication Data

Kendall, Philip C.
  Cognitive-behavioral therapy for impulsive children / by Philip C.
Kendall and Lauren Braswell. — 2nd ed.
    p.   cm.
  Includes bibliographical references and index.
  ISBN 0-89862-013-9
  1. Cognitive therapy for children.   2. Self-control in children.
I. Braswell, Lauren.   II. Title.
  [DNLM: 1. Cognitive Therapy—in infancy & childhood.   2. Cognitive
Therapy—methods.   3. Impulsive Behavior—in infancy & childhood.
WS 350.6 K33c]
RJ505.C63K45   1993
618.92'89142—dc20
DNLM/DLC
for Library of Congress   92-49966
                                                                      CIP

*This book is dedicated to all those children
from whom we have learned so much,
with special thanks to Reed and Mark (P. C. K.)
and Dayna and Will (L. B.).*

Preface

I n 1982, when we decided to undertake the task of writing the first edition of *Cognitive-Behavioral Therapy for Impulsive Children*, we were several years into basic research and clinical work regarding childhood impulsivity and we were concurrently completing a large-scale evaluation of our intervention program (i.e., Kendall & Braswell, 1982b). Three years later, both our program and the appearance of the first edition of this book (Kendall & Braswell, 1985) were sources of encouragement. Now, enthusiasm continues as our program has developed further toward an effective integration of diverse intervention strategies and the inclusion of family and school personnel in the treatment process. For example, Braswell and Bloomquist (1991) have advanced some of the present intervention strategies for application by the families and educators of children with Attention-Deficit Hyperactivity Disorder (ADHD). Kendall has organized training materials for use with the cognitive-behavioral impulsive control program, and this workbook *(Stop and Think)* is now in its second edition (Kendall, 1992a). Indeed, nearly two decades of collective empirical research and clinical application serve as the core of this, the second edition of *Cognitive-Behavioral Therapy for Impulsive Children*.

It is the integration of research and practice that has guided the development of this program from the outset. Hence, it should come as no surprise that the second edition, like the first, is designed for the practitioner who appreciates background research. We offer this book as one that contains not only the actual ins and outs of implementing the program, but also the theory and empirical evidence that support and guide the strategies involved. In the first chapter we outline the guiding theory, describe the nature of cognitive functioning in child and adolescent disorders, and provide a description of a set of attitudes (a therapeutic posture) to steer the therapist. We also state clearly that our program does not require that other interventions be discontinued—quite the contrary, the program for impulse control is very much compatible with other interventions.

Chapters 2 and 3 provide, in different ways, reviews of the background literature. In Chapter 2, studies that evaluate the effects of interventions for impulsive children, both with and without ADHD, with

Conduct Disorder, and with learning disabilities, are reviewed. Studies of the factors that influence outcomes are considered. In Chapter 3, the research literature that addresses the nature of impulsivity is reviewed, again including studies of ADHD, Conduct Disorder, and learning disability, as well as studies of the role of the family in these problem areas.

The methods for proper assessment are reviewed in Chapter 4 and the details of the treatment strategies are described in Chapters 5, 6, and 7. For instance, in Chapter 5 the basic ingredients of the treatment are described, along with transcripts to illustrate their applications. In Chapter 6, the discussion focuses on general strategies for optimizing gains and avoiding pitfalls. Chapter 7 provides a template for guiding intervention with families, teachers, and groups of youth.

Our goal for the second edition, like that of the first, is to provide the information necessary for the implementation of cognitive-behavioral therapy in as competent and thoughtful a manner as possible without more direct training and supervision. More specifically, our goal for the second edition is to provide an updated literature review, an increased focus on the application of the intervention to diverse groups of youth where impulsive control problems are evident, and an expanded sense of the implementation of the program with families and within schools. The reader can now be the judge of whether we have achieved our goals.

Many individuals have contributed to help us to understand impulsivity and many have assisted us in the development, description, application, and evaluation of its treatment. Some have worked with us directly in our respective settings; others have contributed through their correspondence and published articles. Some contributors have been psychologists within the cognitive-behavioral school; others have brought a different perspective to bear on our work. Students, both undergraduate and graduate, and professionals from a diverse areas of training and expertise have provided person-power for our projects and challenged our thinking. Some contributors have been clients and their families, who helped us to hone our recommendations, whereas others, such as our own families and friends, have sparked our continued pursuit of answers to questions. It is to all who have contributed in so many ways that we offer a sincere "thank you."

The reader of this volume, like that of the first edition, will, upon completion of the book, be tempted to tell someone else about the book and its content. Sometimes, a reader will summarize an entire book in just one sentence. To assist such individuals we offer the following: "This book is about how to teach impulsive children to stop and think before they act." We can think of no more accurate or economical summary. Nevertheless, we are willing to wager that the pages that follow add substantially to an understanding of just how the task is accomplished.

Philip C. Kendall
Merion Station, PA
Lauren Braswell
Bloomington, MN

Contents

COGNITIVE-BEHAVIORAL THERAPY
FOR IMPULSIVE CHILDREN

CHAPTER 1

Overview

The principal says to the youth who is appearing in her office, "How do I know that the next time you get teased you won't start hitting again?" The boy of 11 pauses and then looks at the principal and says, "Well, next time someone calls me a name there are lots of things I could do besides hitting. I could laugh—after all, the kid who calls me names, what does he know? And anyway, I will think of what happened the last time—like having to do detention—and I may just walk on by and ignore it." In a separate example, a mother sighs with relief and says, "Son, I'm so glad you came and told me your brother has been changing the TV channels again, instead of just hitting him," and in yet another context a fourth grader thinks to herself, "Wow! I did OK on the social studies test. It did help to read each question real slow and look at all the possible answers before I marked one."

Impossible to achieve? No. Difficult to achieve? Yes, but these three brief vignettes provide examples of the goals toward which cognitive-behavioral therapy for impulsivity is directed. Simply stated, this book is about developing and implementing interventions that teach children to slow down and cognitively examine their behavioral alternatives before acting: in a phrase—to stop and think.

THE COGNITIVE-BEHAVIORAL MODEL

Cognitive-behavioral approaches to the treatment of behavioral, emotional, and academic problems are not restricted to any *one* theoretical tenet or single-minded applied technique. Rather, cognitive-behavioral procedures are a rational amalgam of diverse yet interrelated strategies for providing new learning experiences that involve enactive procedures and a cognitive analysis (see Beck, 1970; Dobson, 1988; Kendall, 1991b; Kendall & Hollon, 1979; Kendall, Vitousek, & Kane, 1992; Mahoney & Arnkoff, 1978; Meichenbaum, 1977). According to the model outlined by Kendall (1985, 1991b), cognitive-behavioral psychotherapy (1) emphasizes both the learning process and the influence of the contingencies and models in the environment, while it (2) underscores the centrality of mediating/information processing factors. The client and therapist work together to think through and behaviorally practice solutions to personal, academic, and interpersonal problems with a consideration of the emotions involved.

As the literature on cognitive-behavioral therapy has grown and its applications broadened, several different themes have emerged. Although there are different applications of the various treatment strategies for specific types of problems, a few principles, in general, serve to guide the cognitive-behavioral therapist, theoretician, and researcher. The following list is adapted from Kendall et al. (1992) and Mahoney (1977b), among others.

1. Cognitive mediational processes are involved in human learning. The human organism responds primarily to cognitive representations of its environment rather than to the environment per se. Children develop these representations as they gain experience with various settings.
2. Thoughts, feelings, and behavior are causally interrelated. Alterations to one aspect of the system will have effects on the other features. Thus, cognitive-behavioral therapy has a strong cognitive–affective–behavioral slant.
3. Cognitive activities, such as preevent expectations, ongoing self-talk, and postevent attributions, are important in understanding psychopathology and producing therapeutic change.
4. Cognitive processes can be cast into testable formulations that are integrated with behavioral paradigms, and it is possible *and* desirable to combine cognitive treatment strategies with behavioral procedures (e.g., modeling, role plays, contingency management).
5. The task of the cognitive-behavioral therapist is to act as a diagnostician, educator, and consultant who assesses maladaptive cognitive processes and works with the client to design learning experiences that may remediate these dysfunctional cognitions and the behavioral and affective patterns with which they correlate.

More specific definitions of the cognitive-behavioral perspective have been offered. Some writers (e.g., Hobbs, Moquin, Tyroler, & Lahey, 1980; Ledwidge, 1978; Wilson, 1978) have placed the cognitive-behavioral approach with behavioral therapy, whereas others (e.g., Beck, Rush, Shaw, & Emery, 1979) prefer to refer to the treatment as cognitive therapy in spite of the several behavioral techniques that are used. Unfortunately, definitional consensus is difficult to locate, for definitions appear to vary in the extent to which they emphasize the cognitive versus the behavioral aspects of this approach to therapy. Urbain and Kendall (1980) proposed that the emphasis on *thinking processes* is the distinguishing feature of cognitive-behavioral approaches with children, but they were quick to add that changes in behavior were the desired outcome. Kendall and Hollon (1979) suggested a balanced emphasis in conceiving the cognitive-behavioral approach as "a purposeful attempt to preserve the demonstrated efficiencies of behavior modification within a less doctrinaire context and to incorporate the cognitive activities of the client in the effort to produce therapeutic change" (p. 1).

At the present juncture, the cognitive-behavioral approach does seem to be chiefly distinguished from the behavioral perspective by the emphasis on cognitive activities, such as beliefs, expectancies, self-statements, and problem solving; yet concern with overt behavior, both in treatment and as an indication of outcome (whether manifested in the use of behavioral contingencies or in explicit skills training), differentiates it from cognitive and insight-oriented approaches.

HISTORICAL INFLUENCES

The definitional variations in emphasis on the cognitive versus behavioral aspects of the cognitive-behavioral perspective grew out of two major historical antecedents: (1) the development of behavioristic interest in the phenomenon of self-control and (2) the emergence of cognitive learning theories of psychotherapy. Skinner wrote about self-control in 1953, yet behaviorists displayed very little interest in the topic until the mid-1960s. Soon, Bandura (1969, 1971) and Kanfer (1970) were exploring behavioral self-control in a series of laboratory studies. In the area of interventions with children, the shift from external to self-regulation was explored with a variety of disorders, but most attention focused on self-regulation of disruptive classroom behavior (e.g., Bolstad & Johnson, 1972, Broden, Hall, & Mitts, 1979; Drabman, Spitalnik, & O'Leary, 1973; Turkewitz, O'Leary, & Ironsmith, 1975). During this transition, behaviorists became desensitized to concepts that acknowledge the complex interrelationship of the organism and its environment and the important role of cognitive information processing in behavioral and emotional adjustment. This shift away from strict stimulus–response (S-R) formulations of human behavior was made explicit in Bandura's *Principles of Behavior Modification* (1969). In this work, Bandura argued for a cognitive–symbolic mechanism governing the basic processes of behavioral change. As Mahoney and Arnkoff (1978) summarized:

> Within a very short period of time cognitive terms and themes became a major aspect of behavioral research. Thus earlier conditioning analyses of self-control began to be replaced by more mediational accounts, and behavior therapists began exploring the relevance of social and cognitive psychology for their clinical endeavors. (p. 692)

The second major historical antecedent, the development of cognitive learning models of psychotherapy, occurred largely outside the domain of strict behavioristic psychology. Two examples of these models are Ellis's (1962) rational–emotive therapy and Beck's (1970, 1976) cognitive therapy. According to Ellis, psychological disturbances are largely the result of illogical, irrational thinking. Such disturbances can be ended if the individual learns to increase rational and to decrease irrational thought. This view assumes that thinking and emotion are integrally related and cannot be entirely separated from each other. In a similar vein, Beck's cognitive therapy, as applied to depression, posits that depression is the result of a negative cognitive set that includes negative beliefs about the self, the world, and the future. The maintenance of these beliefs is the result of distortions in information processing, such as arbitrary inferences or overgeneralizations. Cognitive therapy treats these distortions by assisting the client in testing his/her distorted beliefs. The seminal theories of Ellis and Beck and the procedures following from these theories have had a tremendous impact on psychotherapy—including child and adolescent interventions. Clearly, both Beck and Ellis stress the crucial role of the individual's thoughts or beliefs in the determination of behavior and consider change in these thoughts or beliefs a necessary step in achieving and/or maintaining behavioral change.

CHILD AS CLIENT

Thus far we have outlined the guiding principles, considered definitions and descriptions, and traced a brief history of cognitive-behavioral therapy. These considerations routinely apply to both adult and child applications of cognitive-behavioral strategies. Now, a description of the procedures and their application with children will be highlighted, while noting some of the differences with regard to cognitive-behavioral strategies used with adult clients. It should be noted at the outset that cognitive-behavioral interventions with children are not merely the downward simplification of the approaches used with adults. Rather, children and adolescents differ from adults in important ways, and these differences require alteration in the manner in which the therapist treats the youthful client (see, e.g., Kendall, 1984; Kendall & Williams, 1986).

First, based on the nature of the cognitive problem requiring treatment, a difference was observed between adults and children. Historically, the typical targets of adult cognitive-behavioral therapies were *cognitive errors* (cognitive distortions): irrational beliefs, faulty cognitive processes, misleading internal dialogues. The adult's cognitive errors can also be described as illogical interpretations of the environment, exceedingly high standards for personal performance, and inaccurate perceptions of life's routine demands. Thought processes exist and are active, but the outcomes are faulty. In children, historically, the cognitive problems that were first targeted were *cognitive absences* (cognitive deficiencies): The child does not have or does not employ the cognitive skills needed to perform certain desirable actions. In other terms, the child seemingly fails to engage in the information-processing activities of an effective problem solver and fails to initiate the reflective thinking process that can govern behavior. Initially, then, cognitive distortions were differentiated from cognitive deficiencies as a result of the different targets for treatment for adult versus child clients.

Presently, the distortion–deficiency distinction has a broader application than at its outset. That is, its initial identification was the result of the fact that different disorders in adults and children were those receiving cognitive-behavioral therapy. Adults with depression and anxiety were receiving treatment for distorted thinking, whereas impulsive and hyperactive youth were being trained to overcome cognitive deficiencies. Now, with the more widespread application of integrative cognitive-behavioral therapies, anxious and depressed children, as well as impulsive ones, and angry and aggressive adults, as well as anxious and depressed ones, are involved in cognitive-behavioral therapy. As a result of this growth in application, and based on the research reports of studies that target the identification of cognitive factors in adult and child psychopathology, it seems that the cognitive distortion versus cognitive deficiency distinction has relevance to differentiating several psychological disorders. Individuals with problems of impulse control — be they children or adults — are in need of treatment that provides them with skills to overcome their cognitive deficiencies. They need to learn to employ cognitive strategies to inhibit behavior. Individuals with anxiety and/or depression, both children and adults, need to have their cognitive distortions corrected. They need to learn not to misinterpret their environment and not to see catastrophes and disasters in routine negative outcomes.

In this book we focus on the type of children for whom our cognitive-behavioral treatment is designed: impulsive, non-self-controlled, attention-disordered children. Our program is designed to teach thinking skills to those whose emotional and behavioral problems are linked to acting without thinking. Other types of childhood maladjustment, such as anxiety, isolation, withdrawal, and depression, involve cognitive distortions (errors) and modified applications would be needed (see, for treatment of childhood anxiety disorders, Kendall, Chansky, et al., 1992; for treatment of depression, Stark, Rouse, & Livingston 1991). The distinction between cognitive distortions and cognitive deficiencies has direct implications for treatment (see also Kendall & MacDonald, in press). Unlike therapy with depressed and/or anxious clients, where the therapist has to identify the active but faulty cognitive processes, modify the dysfunctional thinking style, and teach a more adaptive thinking style, the cognitive-behavioral therapist working with impulsive children can proceed more directly to identifying the cognitive absences and teaching the cognitive skills that will help remediate them.

Of course, we do not mean to imply that all client difficulties always fit neatly into this heuristic model of distorted versus deficient thinking processes. For example, after experiencing several years of problematic school functioning, an impulsive acting-out child may become demoralized about his/her lack of academic competence. The child's accurate interpretation of academic woes may lead to more generalized, less accurate beliefs about him/herself. Effective treatment would involve identifying and addressing both problematic aspects of this child's thinking.

As noted earlier, cognitive-behavioral interventions with youth are not identical to those procedures applied to adults. Importantly, given the focus on thinking processes, the therapist must take into account the child's and/or adolescent's level of cognitive development. Many of the cognitive strategies that are appropriate with adult clients cannot be fully understood by children and preschoolers. Some adolescents will be cognitively prepared for more adultlike interventions, but the problem is a genuine one for youngsters. For instance, the confrontation of irrational beliefs, as in rational–emotive therapies, would likely be perceived by a child as a scolding. Not only would the reason for this scolding be unclear, but also the intended outcome — philosophical change — would be somewhat foreign.

Another important distinction between working with children and adults, whatever one's therapeutic approach, is that children do not self-refer for their lack of self-control. We have never had a child call for an appointment in order for us to help him/her overcome impulsivity or hyperactivity. Parents and teachers are typically the adults who decide that the child requires professional treatment. As a result, the therapist is not perceived by the child as a sought-after "helper," as is often true for the help-seeking adult client, but rather is seen as another "teacher" who is likely to "tell me what to do." Special attention must be paid to this inequity in order to ensure that the child comes to perceive the therapeutic experience as enjoyable, if not inviting.

THE POSTURE OF THE THERAPIST

The cognitive-behavioral therapist takes a certain therapeutic posture in his/her interactions with youth. We can describe this posture, or mental attitude, using the terms *consultant, diagnostician,* and *educator.*

We describe a consultant as a therapist who does not have all the answers but who has some ideas that are worth trying out. When functioning as a consusant, the therapist gives the child the opportunity to try something, provides some skills to help evaluate the experience, and aids in the discussion of the merits and demerits of the newly tried skills. A consultant/therapist does not tell the child what to do. Rather, the therapist collaborates with the client to work toward the development of mature problem solving—a goal that cannot be achieved if the therapist tries to solve the problems for the child. In at least three ways—examining behaviors and thinking patterns, trying out new ways of thinking and interacting, and evaluating these new experiences—the therapist collaborates with the child client.

The term *diagnostician* suggests that the therapist gathers and integrates information from a variety of sources. The therapist as diagnostician is an alert and active observer and processor of interactions with the child. Also, the therapist has a great deal of experience and knowledge and can use this background to assist in a formulation of the case. By virtue of this background, the therapist can go beyond the information given: A parent's or teacher's description of the child as impulsive is not sufficient. The description can be more a reflection of the teacher's or parent's misperceptions than the child's misbehavior. Thus, as a diagnostician, the therapist considers the variety of the client's reported difficulties and selects interventions that are consistent with the favored hypothesis.

The third term used to describe the therapist posture is *educator*. As an educator, the therapist helps the child recognize problems, think of alternatives, enact a plan, and make sense of events and the outcomes. Because we are talking about interventions for learning impulse control, we are talking about ways to optimize learning. An active and involved educator will produce the greatest impact on learning. Similarly, an active and involved therapist is preferred. Such a therapist helps arrange learning experiences, participates in these experiences, and provides both negative and positive feedback about the experiences.

THE FOCUS OF THIS SECOND EDITION

The focus of this book is on the treatment of impulsivity. Impulsivity by itself can be detrimental, interfering with a child's capacity to complete important developmental tasks. The impulsive child is likely to have trouble establishing a sence of academic and/or social competence, and, understandably, parents of such children have difficulty trusting the child's capacity for independent functioning.

Impulsivity is one of the three key problems in Attention-Deficit Hyperactivity Disorder (ADHD), plays a role in many learning difficulties, and has been implicated in forms of aggressive acting out. Accordingly, some features of our program apply in interventions for these other related problems. Interested readers are referred to the related programs described by Braswell and Bloomquist (1991) and Hinshaw and Erhardt (1991) for hyperactivity, Wong, Harris, and Graham (1991) for learning problems, and Lochman, White, and Wayland (1991), Kazdin, Bass, Siegel, and Thomas (1989), and Feindler (1991) for aggression and anger.

Our program for the reduction of impulsivity does not require that other interventions be discontinued. That is, concurrent interventions, such as medication for ADHD, are appropriate if not recommended. Indeed, a truly comprehensive intervention for a disorder in which impulsivity plays a central role — such as ADHD — is one that provides parent training, a structured classroom environment with contingency management, possible medication, and individual instruction in impulse control. Whereas the employment of additional treatments is encouraged, we do recommend that the full complement of strategies outlined in this book be implemented in the integrated form that we propose. No single component is sufficient to produce the desired outcomes.

The second edition focuses on the current procedures for the implementation of a cognitive-behavioral intervention for the reduction of impulsivity. As readers of the first edition will notice, there is consistency in the basic components of the treatment we recommend. However, there is greater emphasis placed on (1) the therapist's experience with the problem-solving "posture," (2) the role of the family in the effective treatment of children with problems with impulsivity, and (3) a greater developmental sensitivity, along with (4) recommendations and illustrations for specific materials to be used in the training program. Although, as in the first edition, little discussion has been devoted to topics such as trust, respect, and relationships, these factors are acknowledged as central to any effective therapy. Our program is built on a working relationship between the child and the therapist. Factors that contribute to a strong working relationship are to be encouraged, as are all behavioral patterns that communicate respect and trust.

CHAPTER 2

Background Review

This book really is about how to teach children to "stop and think." We shall explain just what you can do to get children to slow themselves down and examine behavioral alternatives. As part of this process, it is worthwhile first to review what others have done. Accordingly, this chapter reviews the research literature with an eye toward the successes and failures of cognitive-behavioral interventions and the possible factors that moderate these differences in outcome.

Several changes in this chapter since the first edition are worthy of note. In the first edition, we detailed a large number of treatment outcome studies with subjects selected by test-based research criteria as well as those presenting with clinically significant problems. In the current edition we have shortened the discussion of some of the specific studies and summarized more across groups of studies—we have endeavored to provide more discussion of the most recent research. We have retained detailed descriptions of selected efforts, including the studies that were central to the development of the intervention presented in this book. In addition, in the first edition, we organized our discussion according to the type of intervention (e.g., self-instructional training vs. problem-solving training). Over the past few years, however, these approaches have been increasingly combined. Thus, although we discuss the diverse historical influences leading to the development of these approaches, it seems most appropriate to view them as variations on a common theme. In the current volume, the discussion of the outcome literature is organized around the type of disorder that is addressed by the intervention (e.g., ADHD behavior, Conduct Disorder behavior, or learning difficulties) making this chapter consistent with the new organization in the chapter on the nature of the disorder. The current review focuses largely on externalizing disorders and learning difficulties. Readers interested in outcome research with internalizing forms of childhood disorder are referred to the works of Kendall, Chansky, et al. (1992) and Stark et al. (1991).

DEVELOPMENT OF COGNITIVE-BEHAVIORAL APPROACHES WITH EXTERNALIZING CHILDREN

There have been several specific influences on the cognitive-behavioral literature dealing with children. First, an early form of self-instructional training came on the scene (Meichenbaum & Goodman, 1971). Accordingly, the factors that led to the self-instructional procedures are themselves important factors in the development of cognitive-behavioral therapy in general. Second, the focus on problem solving as a form of prevention and treatment had an impressive impact on the field of child clinical psychology. The antecedents of problem solving are therefore also relevant to the development of cognitive-behavioral procedures with children struggling with various forms of acting-out behavior.

Self-Instructional Training

In addition to the historical–theoretical underpinnings of cognitive-behavioral approaches cited in Chapter 1, Meichenbaum (1979b) and Craighead (1982) highlighted areas of theorizing and research that contributed specifically to the development of self-instructional training. The first and most significant influence that these authors highlighted was the study of the functional relationship between language and behavior that occurred within the field of child development. The most frequently cited examples are the theories of Soviet psychologists Luria (1959, 1961) and Vygotsky (1962, 1987; see also Meichenbaum, 1977).

Vygotsky proposed that the internalization of verbal commands is the crucial step in a child's establishment of voluntary control over behavior. Luria, Vygotsky's student, elaborated a developmental theory of verbal control that focuses on two interrelated developmental shifts. One shift concerns the origin and nature of the speech that does the controlling. Luria suggested a sequence in which the child's behavior is initially controlled by the verbalizations of others, usually adults (other-external). In the next stage, the child's own overt verbalizations direct his/her behavior (self-external), and finally, by age 5 or 6, the child's behavior is controlled by his/her own covert self-verbalizations (self-internal). The second type of shift or change concerns the type of control provided by these verbalizations. Luria theorized that during the other-external and self-external phases verbal control is primarily impulsive rather than semantic. Impulsive control refers to speech as a physical stimulus that can inhibit or disinhibit responses. As the child develops, the type of control shifts to semantic, with the child learning to respond to speech as a carrier of specific symbolic meaning. As a result of these two shifts, by approximately age 6, the normally developing child acquires self-internal regulating speech and is responsive to the content of verbalizations.

Mussen (1963) has also argued for a sequential model of development of verbal control of behavior that is very similar to that of Luria and Vygotsky, and other investigators have obtained results supportive of such a progression in normally developing children (Berk, 1986; Bivens & Berk, 1990; Lovaas, 1964; Bem, 1967). This work, along with that of Meacham (1978) and Rondal (1976), does suggest, however, that the age ranges in which the different types of verbal control are demonstrated may vary with the nature of the behavioral task. In a review of theories and studies of private speech, Kohlberg, Yaeger, and Hjentholm (1968) emphasized the importance of private speech in self-initiated regulation and direction of ongoing overt motor behavior. However, this view of the role of private speech is not without its critics. Flavell (1977) objected to interpreting the source of self-control as exclusively verbal, pointing to the importance of nonverbal control via gestures and environmental manipulations. Works by Zivin (1979) and Copeland (1983) review the developmental significance of children's talking to themselves. More recently, Berk and Potts (1991) have presented data that support the view that children with attentional difficulties may lag behind normally developing children in their use of the most mature forms of covert self-speech, but this delay may be more the *result* of their poorly functioning attentional regulation system rather than the *cause* of such attentional difficulties. Although these findings are preliminary, they suggest that the relationship between self-speech and attention to task may be bidirectional (e.g., task-relevant self-talk and attentional functioning influence each other) rather than unidirectional (e.g., task-oriented self-talk leads to better on-task behavior). In the past, Lurian formulations of verbal self-regulation, whatever their shortcomings, have served as the theoretical bases for self-instructional interventions.

The second influence noted by Meichenbaum was research on the child's self-mediated cognitive strategies, such as the work of Mischel and his colleagues on delay of gratification. In a 1974 review, Mischel summarized evidence that self-generated strategies, such as self-instructions and self-praise, helped children reduce frustration during delay-of-gratification tasks. In this type of research, the "training" in self-instruction is very brief; in fact, it usually involves the experimenter's simply instructing the child to say a particular sentence or think a particular thought. Patterson and Mischel also examined verbal self-control in a series of studies on verbal strategies for resisting distraction (Mischel & Patterson, 1976; Patterson & Mischel, 1976). The findings suggested that preschoolers do not spontaneously produce self-instructions to help them cope with highly distracting stimuli, but when provided with a specific cognitive plan the children are able to work longer in the distracting situation. Very similar research strategies have also been utilized in studies of rule-following behavior (Monohan & O'Leary, 1971; O'Leary, 1968), with results suggesting that verbalization of simple self-instructions can reduce rule breaking in children.

While the findings of these two different areas of research are basically complementary, different styles or methods of training in self-
instructions have followed from these approaches. In an effort to bring
clarity and organization to this body of research, studies in which training
resembles that employed in delay of gratification and resistance to distraction research are termed *noninteractive*, for training involves the experimenter's merely telling the child what to do or say. Studies that reflect
more of the influence of Luria's stage theory approach are labeled *interactive* or *elaborated*, for training involves more child–experimenter exchange and interaction in the process of the training for self-instruction. A
subgroup of studies within the interactive category employs self-
instructional procedures, but this training is provided within the context of
more operant formulations of self-control. In these studies, self-
instruction is taught as a skill along with other skills such as self-
monitoring, self-evaluation, and self-reinforcement.

Most recent research has involved the more elaborated form of
self-instructional training. Elaborated or interactive self-instructional
training considers self-instructions important in building cognitive sche-
mata that are capable of guiding, directing, and coordinating other aspects
of self-regulatory behavior. The prototype for these studies was conducted
by Meichenbaum and Goodman (1971) and elaborated by Kendall and
Finch (1979b). As described by Meichenbaum (1975, 1977), in the first
stage of training the therapist or tutor models the behaviors associated
with successful task performance while talking to him/herself out loud.
These verbalizations of self-instructions relate to the specifics of the task
and include statements of problem definition (i.e., clarifying and understanding the exact requirements of the task at hand), problem approach
(planning a general strategy for solving the problem), focusing attention,
selecting an answer, and self-reinforcing for correct performance or using
a coping statement for incorrect performance. After observing the therapist perform several tasks, children perform a task while talking to themselves out loud. Usually at this point the therapist assists the child in
remembering to employ the modeled sequence of self-verbalizations. The
therapist and the child typically alternate performing tasks, and as they
proceed through a task, the therapist gradually fades these verbalizations
to a whisper and encourages the child to do the same. Eventually, the
therapist and child self-instruct covertly, using the internalized statements
to control and direct task performance. Thus, self-instructional procedures include training in the use of task-directing verbalizations, self-
reinforcing statements, and modeling of task-appropriate behavior. The
effectiveness of this strategy, often as part of a more comprehensive
program, has been evaluated with cognitively impulsive children as well as

with aggressive, hyperactive, non-self-controlled, and behavior-problem children.

Problem-Solving Approaches

A second major class of interventions within the cognitive-behavioral realm emphasizes a problem-solving approach to social and interpersonal difficulties. In terms of historical influences, Jahoda (1953, 1958) is frequently cited as one of the first to suggest that the ability to solve real-life interpersonal problems is one criterion of mental health. The 1970s witnessed a series of attempts to formulate problem solving as a set of skills relevant for clinical endeavors. Interpreting problem solving within a behavioral framework, D'Zurilla and Goldfried (1971) defined it as "a *behavioral process . . . which* (a) *makes available a variety of potentially effective response alternatives for dealing with the problematic situation and* (b) *increases the probability of selecting the most effective response from among these various alternatives*" (p. 108) (emphasis in original). D'Zurilla and Goldfried went on to outline five stages of problem solving, including general orientation, problem definition and formulation, generation of alternatives, decision making, and verification.

Mahoney (1977a) described a seven-step problem-solving sequence. The stages he elaborated include specification of problem; collection of information; identification of causes; examination of options; narrowing of options and experimentation; comparison of data; and extension, revision, or replacement of the solution. Spivack, Shure, Platt, and their associates at Hahnemann University Mental Health Center (Shure & Spivack, 1978; Spivack, Platt, & Shure, 1976; Spivack & Shure, 1974) have theorized that effective interpersonal cognitive problem solving requires the subskills of sensitivity to human problems, the ability to generate alternative solutions, the conceptualization of the appropriate means to achieve a given solution, and a sensitivity to consequences and cause–effect relationships in human behavior. These three systems evidence a high degree of similarity and, perhaps, reflect the beginnings of a consensus on the nature of interpersonal problem solving.

The Hahnemann research group has studied the nature of the relationship between these skills and overt social adjustment. Positive relationships between these Interpersonal Cognitive Problem-Solving (ICPS) skills and adjustment have been demonstrated in 4- and 5-year-olds (Shure & Spivack, 1970; Shure, Spivack, & Jaeger, 1971; Spivack & Shure, 1974), 10-year-olds (Larcen, Spivack, & Shure, 1972), adolescents (Platt, Spivack, Altman, Altman, & Peizer, 1974; Spivack & Levine, 1963), and adults (Platt & Spivack, 1972a, 1972b, 1973). It should be noted, however, that negligible relationships with adjustment were reported in a study of 6- to 11-year-old children from a normal school and with IQ controlled (Kendall & Fischler, 1984). In the Kendall and Fischler (1984) study, ICPS skills were scored quantitatively, as suggested by Spivack and Shure (1974). Significant relationships between problem solving and adjustment were found, however, when the skills were scored according to variations in the *quality* of the children's solutions (Fischler & Kendall, 1988). In relating their positive findings to the development of a training program, Spivack and Shure (1974) state their hypothesis as "one should be able to enhance the personal adjustment of young children if one can enhance their ability to see a human problem, their appreciation of different ways of handling it, and their sensitivity to the potential consequences of what they do" (p. 21).

The problem-solving approaches to intervention involve training children in the specific components of effective problem solving. For example, most programs are designed to teach the components of problem solving: (1) initial inhibition of impulsive responses ("stop and think"); (2) problem identification (ways to recognize problems were discussed and children shared problems within the group); (3) generating alternatives ("brainstorming"); (4) evaluating consequences ("think ahead"); (5) making a plan; and (6) evaluating the effectiveness of the initially chosen solution and selecting a backup plan. Some problem-solving training programs also include content addressing social perspective-taking skills such as (1) increasing awareness of feelings; (2) developing social–causal reasoning; and (3) increasing awareness of the perspective of others.

It is important to note that several studies have examined the impact of social problem-solving training with a focus on the prevention of childhood disorder. For example, Weissberg et al. (1981) examined the effects of intensive social problem-solving training with suburban and inner-city third graders. The intervention was found to be effective with the suburban children but not with the urban children. The interested reader can examine the impact of such preventive programs with "normal" children in a number of other investigations (Allen, Chinsky, Larcen, Lochman, & Selinger, 1976; Feldhusen & Houtz, 1975; McClure, Chinsky, & Larcen, 1978; Stone, Hinds, & Schmidt, 1975).

OUTCOME STUDIES ADDRESSING ADHD-TYPE BEHAVIOR

A large number of studies have implemented variations of cognitive-behavioral therapy with children manifesting inattention, impulsivity, and hyperactivity. Due to controversy over construct validity, our discussion distinguishes among those studies that select subjects primarily by test performance on specific measures, by teacher identification as manifesting inattentive and/or impulsive behavior, and by parental identification as manifesting clinically significant levels of disturbance.

Test-Selected Subjects

Some self-instructional intervention studies have identified their samples solely on the basis of cognitive impulsivity as defined as task performance on a measure such as the Matching Familiar Figures (MFF) test (Kagan, Rosman, Day, Albert, & Phillips, 1964). This measure is a match-to-sample task in which the child's latency to first response and the number of incorrect responses are recorded. Typically a child is judged impulsive if his/her latency is below and reponse errors are above the respective medians of a same-aged sample. The MFF is also frequently used as an outcome measure, and some evidence for a relationship between cognitive and behavioral impulsivity does exist (see review by Messer, 1976; Egeland, Bielke, & Kendall, 1980); however, there is controversy over the construct validity of this measure (Bentler & McClain, 1976; Block, Block, & Harrington, 1974; Kagan & Messer, 1975; Messer, 1976). Given this controversy, studies using only the MFF or similar measures of cognitive impulsivity for case identification will be discussed separately from investigations using more "clinical" criteria such as parent or teacher referral. The reader is also referred to the discussion of the construct of impulsivity presented in Chapter 3.

Meichenbaum and Goodman's prototype self-instructional training (1971, Study II) used MFF-selected kindergarten and first-grade subjects in an examination of the efficacy of the cognitive self-instructional training relative to a modeling-only and control group. The self-instructional training condition employed the procedures just described; the modeling condition was identical to the self-instructional condition except for the absence of any verbal self-instructions. Relative to the control group, both treatment groups demonstrated significant increases in response latency following four 30-minute training sessions, but only the self-instructional group obtained a decrease in errors. This finding suggests that self-instructions do have an impact beyond that obtained simply by modeling successful task behavior. Abikoff (1979) has suggested that the results of this study are qualified by the high degree of overlap between the test, the MFF, and the picture-matching materials used in training. This critique does have relevance for evaluating the overall level of improved performance, but the overlap between training and test materials does not necessarily qualify the contrast between the self-instructional and modeling conditions.

Other investigations involving test-selected impulsive subjects have tended to achieve positive results in terms of modifying impulsive response style on specific paper-and-pencil measures, particularly when self-instructions include a self-reinforcement component (Bender, 1976; Cohen, Meyers, Schlesser, & Rodick, 1982; Kendall & Finch, 1978; Nelson & Birkimer, 1978; Wright, 1973). The results of Cullinan, Epstein, and Silver (1977) suggest, however, that even these modest changes cannot be achieved if the treatment is too brief or involves only videotaped rather than live modeling and/or if subjects are not required to use the self-verbalizations while actually solving problems.

Teacher-Identified Subjects

Another large subgroup of studies with children exhibiting ADHD behavior includes subjects selected on the basis of teacher reports of impulsive, inattentive, and/or overactive behavior in the classroom. This target population seems likely to manifest greater difficulty than may be the case with subjects identified solely on the basis of performance on a single measure of impulsivity but who, as a group, present with less extreme behavioral issues than would be expected with a sample of children who all meet formal criteria for a diagnosis such as ADHD.

In an effort to apply their theoretical formulations of the problem-solving process, Spivack and Shure (1974) developed a training program to be used by preschool teachers for instructing children in ICPS skills. This intervention was implemented with 113 preschool children who had been teacher classified as impulsive, inhibited, or adjusted. The program included dialogues, games, and activities for the teacher to use with the children in a series of 46 daily lessons, each lasting approximately 20 minutes. The early sessions focused on developing what Spivack and Shure believe to be prerequisites for problem-solving skills, such as the ability to identify and discriminate emotions. Later sessions taught alternative, consequential, and means–ends thinking as applied to interpersonal problem situations. At posttreatment the experimental subjects demonstrated significant improvement in generation of alternative solutions and consequential thinking relative to the no-treatment controls. Improvement on the teacher ratings of behavior was also noted, but the teachers were not blind to the treatment status of the children. At 1-year follow-up, teachers who were not informed of the children's treatment status also rated the trained subjects better adjusted than the controls.

These results are extremely interesting, but the absence of an attention control group, particularly given the lengthy nature of treatment, makes it difficult to rule out alternative explanations of change. In fact, Sharp (1981) and Rickel, Eshelman, and Loigman (1983) were unsuccessful in their attempt to replicate the Spivack and Shure findings while controlling for the previously noted methodological problems. The efforts of Sharp (1981) and Rickel et al. (1983) did not, however, constitute an exact replication, because the training was conducted by graduate students outside the classroom rather than by the children's actual preschool teachers. As noted by Urbain and Savage (1989), using the classroom teacher as trainer may be a particularly important component in helping young children learn to use the skills in real-world settings since the trainer's presence would presumably function as a cue to prompt skill usage.

In a variation on their original curriculum in which the teacher provides the training, Shure and Spivack (1978) have also reported success with a program in which the mothers of preschoolers were trained to conduct the intervention with their own children. Forty mother–child pairs were selected on the basis of the child's demonstrating overly impulsive or overly inhibited behavior in the preschool setting and being low on measures of the ICPS skills. Each mother administered the program games and dialogues at home with her child for 20 minutes a day over a 3-month period. On the ICPS tests, the experimental children improved significantly more than did the untrained, matched controls in their ability to generate alternative solutions and demonstrate consequential thinking. There were no significant changes in sensitivity to the existence of an interpersonal problem, and the authors suggest that this skill could be too developmentally advanced for the average preschool child. Also, the trained children did not differ from the control children at posttest on measures of impersonal thinking skills, indicating that treatment effects were specific to interpersonal thinking skills. At pretest, 17 of the 20 experimental children were rated as not adjusted by their teachers, but at posttest only 5 were still so rated. In contrast, 16 of 20 controls were rated as not adjusted at pretest, and posttest ratings indicated 11 of the 20 remained not adjusted.

Interview data from the mothers suggested that the trained mothers changed their problem-solving style in dealing with their children as a result of exposure to the program. The mothers also demonstrated significantly improved means–ends thinking at posttreatment. In terms of mother–child outcomes, the children's significantly improved alternative thinking abilities were correlated with both the mothers' improved childrearing style and increased means–ends thinking scores. The mothers' means–ends thinking scores were also related to the children's improvement in consequential thinking. The research of Spivack, Shure, and their colleagues demonstrates many laudable features, such as regular analyses for possible sex differences, explicit examination of the link between changes in ICPS skills and change in behavior, and a generally programmatic approach to their topic of study. Unfortunately, their failure to utilize proper control conditions makes it difficult to rule out competing explanations, such as the possible effects of a consistent increase in maternal attention and mother–child interaction, whatever the nature of this interaction. Also, while the authors provide beautifully detailed descriptions of the intervention, evaluation procedures are rather loosely described, making accurate replication quite difficult.

Working from a perspective that emphasizes an operant view of self-control, Cameron and Robinson (1980) evaluated a training program that emphasized both self-instructional procedures and other self-management strategies. The subjects were four 7- to 8-year-old children selected by their teachers as demonstrating academic and behavior problems. Using a multiple-baseline, across-individuals design, the authors assessed on-task behavior during math class, math performance in terms of percent accurate, and self-correction rate in reading. Each child received 12 individual 30-minute sessions over 3 weeks. Self-instructional training procedures were applied to math problems and additional training was provided in self-monitoring and self-reinforcement for correct performance. The training resulted in significant increases in on-task behavior for two of the three children, and all three showed gains in math accuracy. Training did seem to generalize to reading, but the authors cautioned that factors such as the nature of the reading program and simple maturation might also explain the improved reading. These findings provide support for self-instructional plus other self-regulation skills as a method of improving on-task behavior and academic performance in specific subject areas.

As previously stated, Meichenbaum and Goodman's (1971) research used an elaborate, interactive form of training. In Study I, the subjects were second-grade children who were teacher identified as hyperactive or lacking in self-control and randomly assigned to cognitive training, attention control, or assessment control conditions. Subjects in the experimental and attention control groups received four 30-minute training sessions with both groups using the same training tasks but only the experimental group being taught self-instructions. Two types of dependent measures were employed. Task performance measures included the Porteus Maze test, the MFF, and the Picture Arrangement (PA), Block Design (BD), and Coding subtests of the Wechsler Intelligence Scale for Children (WISC) (Wechsler, 1949). Measures of classroom behavior included behavioral observations and a teacher questionnaire designed to assess the child's level of self-control. Posttesting indicated that the self-instructional group improved significantly more than the two control groups on MFF latency and WISC PA and Coding subtests. Both the self-instructional and attention control groups made significantly fewer qualitative errors on the Porteus than did the assessment control group. The pattern of relatively positive results was basically maintained at 4-

week follow-up. However, the classroom measures revealed no significant group differences for the behavioral observations or teacher ratings of classroom behavior. Self-instructions seemed to improve task performance on certain tests, but, perhaps because of the limited number of sessions or the nature of the training materials, generalization to classroom behavior did not occur.

Numerous case studies and group treatment studies have followed and many have sought to develop improved methods for attaining this elusive generalization. After a successful case study (Kendall & Finch, 1976) and group outcome study with test-identified subjects (Kendall & Finch, 1978), Kendall and colleagues initiated a series of studies with teacher-referred subjects in an effort to clarify features of self-instructional training that affect its impact and generalizability.

Kendall and Wilcox (1980) examined the contribution of different types of self-instructions to the achievement of generalized change. This study compared self-instructional training that focuses on the specific training task (concrete labeling) with training that was relevant to the task but was also general and could thus be applied to other situations (conceptual labeling). The 33 8- to 12-year-old teacher-referred subjects were assigned to one of two treatment conditions or an attention control group using a randomized block procedure, with teachers' blind Self-Control Rating Scale (SCRS) ratings as the blocking factor. All subjects were seen for six 40-minute sessions, but only the two treatment groups received self-instructional training with modeling and a response-cost contingency. The training materials for sessions 1 through 4 were psychoeducational tasks, and in sessions 5 and 6 training focused on interpersonal play situations that required cooperation. At posttest and 1-month follow-up, teachers' blind ratings of self-control and hyperactivity evidenced significant change due to treatment, with the treatment effects stronger for the conceptual labeling group. Thus, generalization of treatment effects to the classroom was found. A self-report measure of impulsivity showed no change, and all three groups improved on the MFF and Porteus Mazes. In addition, Kendall and Wilcox provided data on the self-control ratings of nonreferred children to give some guidelines or norms for assessing treatment impact (see also Kendall & Norton-Ford, 1982b, and Kendall & Grove, 1988, for more detailed discussion of the methods of normative comparisons). At posttreatment and follow-up, the conceptual treatment group fell within one standard deviation of the mean for the nonreferred children (see also Thackwray, Meyers, Schlesser, & Cohen, 1985).

At 1-year follow-up (Kendall, 1981b), numerous improvements were found for subjects in all treatment groups—perhaps due to increased age. Teacher ratings showed differences favoring the conceptually trained children, but with a small number of children available, the differences did not reach statistical significance. However, it was found that conceptually trained children showed significantly better recall of the material they had learned than either the concrete or the control group. Conceptually trained children were rated by their new classroom teachers as not sufficiently lacking in self-control to warrant referral. Although the documentation of long-term effects was not compelling, there was a suggestive pattern of relationships between the age of the subject and long-term maintenance of gains.

In a study of the relative effectiveness of individual and group application of the cognitive-behavioral intervention procedures, Kendall and Zupan (1981) employed twice as many treatment sessions (12) as had Kendall and Wilcox (1980). Thirty teacher-referred, non-self-controlled classroom problem children from grades 3 to 5 were assigned according to a randomized block procedure to either the individual treatment condition, the group treatment condition, or a nonspecified group treatment (control) condition. Except for the instructions relating to the cognitive-behavioral self-control training proper, children in all three conditions were given similar tasks, task instructions, and performance feedback; however, only the children in either the individual or the group self-control conditions received training in the cognitive-behavioral strategies.

Multiple-method assessments were used to evaluate treatment procedures, including measures of children's task performance and cognitive skills and two teacher ratings (teachers blind to treatment conditions) of classroom behavior. In addition to children's performance (latencies and errors) on the MFF, two tasks for assessing cognitive interpersonal skills were utilized: the Means–Ends Problem Solving (MEPS) task (Shure & Spivack, 1972) and Chandler's (1973) bystander cartoons (measure of social perspective taking). Teachers who were blind to subjects' conditions completed the SCRS and Conners hyperactivity index. Each of these assessment measures was administered pretreatment, posttreatment, and at 2-month follow-up. The Peabody Picture Vocabulary Test (PPVT) (Dunn, 1965) was administered pretreatment to acquire a general index of each child's intellectual abilities.

The most striking gains were seen in pretreatment to posttreatment changes on the teachers' blind ratings (i.e., SCRS and hyperactivity). Analysis of the teachers' blind ratings of self-control indicated that the children in the group and individual treatment conditions demonstrated significant improvements that were significantly superior to the changes in the nonspecific treatment condition. These findings provide evidence of the generalized effects of the treatment to classroom behavior. The changes in teachers' ratings of hyperactivity parallel somewhat the self-control ratings; however, the changes were significant for all three treatment conditions. Analysis of maintenance effects indicated that both self-control and hyperactivity ratings showed significant improvements, but that the improvement at follow-up was independent of the child's treatment condition.

Improvements that were independent of the child's treatment condition were seen in performance on the MFF. However, while changes in MFF latency scores were not maintained at follow-up, improvements in MFF errors were. That is, when MFF latencies and errors are considered together, the results indicated that children were performing in a somewhat fast and accurate manner, a style that is more desirable than either the fast, inaccurate (impulsive) or slow, accurate (reflective) style. Changes in perspective taking at follow-up were positive. Both individual and group treatments produced lasting improvements; the nonspecific control condition did not. Changes in MEPS test performance were in the opposite direction from what would be expected. This trend was likely the result of the use of the same test material for repeated administration and the tendency of the children to tell shorter stories on each administration. Shorter stories resulted in lower MEPS scores.

It should be noted, however, that significant improvements across the assessment periods for children in all three groups were not surprising. The nonspecific (group treatment) control condition was included to control for the effects of group participation; it was intended as an attention-placebo condition in a group context. Because of the problems that arose in the control group of non-self-controlled children, therapists eventually employed reprimands, forceful comments, and other group control techniques to maintain order. As a result of these procedures and the children's response to the training materials, some minor gains were expected.

In terms of normative comparisons (Kendall & Grove, 1988) using the teachers' blind-ratings data, the mean SCRS scores of the cognitive-behavioral treatment conditions at posttreatment were within one standard deviation of the normative mean. Similarly, the hyperactivity ratings for the cognitive-behavioral treatment conditions were brought within the normative range. These normative comparisons suggest that the children receiving the cognitive-behavioral treatment (individually or in groups) evidenced improvements that brought them (at posttreatment) within a normal range of self-control and hyperactivity. These improvements, resulting from lengthier treatments, were greater than those reported in Kendall and Wilcox (1980).

At 1-year follow-up (Kendall, 1982b), improvements were found for subjects across treatment conditions. Only the children receiving group treatment were not significantly different from nonproblem children on ratings of self-control; only the children receiving individual treatment were not significantly different from nonproblem children on hyperactivity ratings. Structured interviews indicated that individually treated children showed significantly better recall of the ideas they had learned and produced significantly more illustrations of use of the ideas than children in either the group treatment or the nonspecific treatment conditions. Apparently, there was evidence for generalization to the classroom (as evident in the teachers' ratings) but an absence of compelling evidence for long-term maintenance.

Considering the hypothesized importance of behavioral contingencies within the comprehensive cognitive training program, Kendall and Braswell (1982b) compared the efficacy of an intervention involving self-instructional training with response-cost contingencies, role plays, and modeling with an intervention utilizing *only* the behavioral techniques (modeling, response-cost contingencies, and role plays, but no cognitive training). Twenty-seven non-self-controlled problem children (8 to 12 years old) were randomly assigned to the cognitive-behavioral treatment, the behavioral-only treatment, or the attention control group. All children received 12 sessions of individual therapist contact focusing on psychoeducational, play, and interpersonal tasks and situations. The children receiving the cognitive-behavioral intervention improved teachers' blind ratings of self-control, and both the cognitive-behavioral and behavioral treatments improved teachers' blind ratings of hyperactivity. Parent ratings did not show that treatment produced behavioral improvement in the home setting. Several performance measures (cognitive style, academic achievement) showed improvements for the cognitive-behavioral and behavioral conditions, whereas only the cognitive-behavioral treatment improved children's self-reported self-concept. Naturalistic observations in the classroom showed significant variability, but off-task verbal and off-task physical behaviors showed some decrease in frequency as a result of both of the treatments. Some of these improvements were maintained at 10-week follow-up for the cognitive-behavioral condition; however, 1-year follow-up data did not show significant differences across conditions. Despite its strengths, this study can be faulted for not implementing the behavioral condition in a manner that would be endorsed by most behaviorists. Few behaviorists would expect contingencies used only in the training setting and not in the environment targeted for change (in this case the classroom) to have much impact on behavior in the target environment without careful planning for generalization. In more recent years, in fact, both those advocating traditional behavioral approaches and those aligned with cognitive-behavioral methods have stressed the need to provide training, or at least prompts, for skill use in the targeted environment (Stokes & Osnes, 1989; Kendall, 1989). The results of Kendall and Braswell (1982b) argue for the effectiveness of the combined cognitive and behavioral components of the intervention but highlight the difficulty in achieving durable behavioral improvement, particularly in the absence of well-elaborated training for generalization.

Studies with Children Meeting Criteria for ADHD

While the findings of studies with test-identified and teacher-referred subjects were largely supportive of the view that cognitive-behavioral intervention could lead to at least some degree of improvement, applications with subjects meeting clinical criteria for the psychiatric diagnosis of ADHD have constituted a more challenging test for these intervention methods.

Considering those interventions that placed a greater relative emphasis on self-instructions, the early reports of successful treatment of hyperactive children using even very brief, noninteractive forms of self-instructional training led to a sense of promise concerning the use of these methods with this population (Bornstein & Quevillon, 1976; Palkes, Stewart, & Kahana, 1968). Unfortunately, later attempts to replicate these findings were not always successful (Friedling & O'Leary, 1979; Palkes, Stewart, & Freedman, 1972).

Other investigators have examined the impact of more elaborate, lengthy versions of this type of training. In one of the most comprehensive early efforts, Douglas, Parry, Marton, and Garson (1976) employed self-instructional procedures with hyperactive boys. To be included in the study, the child's parents and his teacher had to agree that the child demonstrated symptoms of hyperactivity, such as attentional problems, excessive motor activity level, and impulsivity. In addition, the child had to be rated above the cutoff score on the Conners Parent and Teacher Rating Scales for Hyperactivity and demonstrate a mean latency of less than 10 seconds on the MFF. All subjects were from upper-lower-class or middle-class homes, and no child with an IQ below 80 was included. Subjects ranged in age from 6 years, 1 month to 10 years, 11 months. The experimental group included 18 subjects, and the control group contained 11, with groups not differing on age, IQ, and Conners score. Training involved two 1-hour sessions per week for 12 weeks. Self-instructional procedures were applied to a broad range of training materials, including the child's actual homework and interpersonal problem situations. In addition, a minimum of 12 consultation sessions with each child's parents and six sessions with classroom teachers were held. These sessions explained the training to parents and teachers and provided instructions in the implementation of self-instructional procedures at home and at school. On occasion, parents or teachers observed and participated in the child's training session.

Treatment impact was assessed via an extensive test battery, including the MFF, Porteus Mazes, Story Completion Test (Parry, 1973), Bender

Visual-Motor Gestalt Test (Bender, 1938), memory tests from the Detroit Tests of Learning Aptitude (Baker & Leland, 1967), Durrell Analysis of Reading Difficulty (Durrell, 1955), the Wide Range Achievement Test (Jastak, Bijou, & Jastak, 1965), and the parent and teacher versions of the Conners.

At posttest, the treatment group showed significant improvement over its pretreatment performance on 9 of 10 task performance measures, whereas the control group showed significant improvement on only 1 measure. The treatment group did not show improvement on either the parent or the teacher behavior ratings. At 3-month follow-up, the treatment group maintained its improved level on 8 of 10 measures, and the control group maintained its one improved score. As the authors point out, improvements were observed in the treatment group on measures that were not the specific focus of training, such as the reading and Story Completion tests. The lack of significant change on the Conners scale indicated a lack of generalization of treatment effects to the home or school setting. The lack of generalization is troubling given the authors' reported attempts to involve parents and teachers in the training process; however, there was no assessment of the extent to which the parents or teachers actually used or prompted the child's use of the methods in the home and school environments. In addition, there was no explicit program of behavioral contingencies to accompany either the training of self-instructional procedures or the use of these methods at home or school. The Douglas et al. (1976) investigation can be credited for careful subject selection and thorough assessment of treatment effects. The lack of impact on home or school behavior is disappointing, but the results do support the efficacy of self-instructional training for producing lasting improvement in performance on certain cognitive and visual–motor tests.

In a study of the role of expectations and the differential effectiveness of external versus internal monitoring, Bugental, Whalen, and Henker (1977) provided treatment for 36 7- to 12-year-old hyperactive and impulsive boys, half of whom were receiving methylphenidate. Treatment was conducted twice a week for 8 weeks, with the experimenter/tutors utilizing either self-instructional training or contingent social reinforcement. Both interventions were aimed at increasing the child's attention and correct performance on academic tasks. The results indicated that children whose attributional styles were congruent with their treatment (high personal control/self-control training or high external control/social contingency management) achieved better Porteus scores than those in noncongruent combinations. Also, self-instructional training was more effective with nonmedicated children, whereas external control was superior with the medicated subjects. As Bugental et al. (1977) stated, "Change strategies (behavioral management, educational programs, psychotherapy, medical intervention) have implicit attributional textures which interact with the attributional network of the individual to influence treatment impact" (p. 881). Thus, children who were already somewhat internal in their attributional styles responded more positively to an internally oriented intervention whereas an externally managed intervention proved to be most effective with children manifesting external attributional styles. Unfortunately, neither intervention produced changes on a teacher rating scale. Bugental, Collins, Collins, and Chaney (1978) carried out a 6-month follow-up with these children. Subjects receiving self-instructional training had increased their perceptions of personal control; however, according to teacher ratings, the social contingency group had changed in the direction of reduced hyperactivity. All subjects improved their performance on the Porteus Mazes. The authors suggested, consistent with our position, that the ideal intervention might be some *combination* of self-control procedures and social contingencies.

The use of problem-solving training with severely hyperactive boys was examined by Kirmil-Gray, Duckham-Shoor, and Thoresen (1980). Eight hyperactive boys, ages 7 to 10 years, currently on stimulant medication, were selected to participate in this intervention via rigorous diagnostic procedures. The intervention had two components: problem-solving training for the children and behavioral management training for the parents. The problem-solving training involved 48 sessions designed to teach social problem solving as well as motor inhibition, attending behavior, and self-direction skills. Each 45-minute session included explanation, modeling, role playing, and game playing. During training, a reinforcement system was operational in order to reward the child for appropriate behavior and use of new skills. The parent training in behavioral management involved eight 2- to 3-hour sessions in which parents received instruction in implementing behavioral techniques with their children. The children's teachers were also provided consultation on the behavioral management of hyperactive children. Four subjects received both the problem-solving and parent training interventions, two received only parent training, and the remaining two were assessment controls. An individualized medication reduction schedule was developed for each of the six treatment subjects, with the goal for all being complete medication withdrawal by the end of training. All subjects were observed over an 18-week period, including 3 to 4 weeks of baseline, 12 weeks of treatment, and 2 weeks of follow-up. Both disruptive behavior and social interactions were observed. Assessment methods included direct observations in the classroom, teacher and parent reports of behavior, and numerous task performance measures.

The basic findings from these multiple-outcome measures indicated that acceptable behavior was maintained with the complete withdrawal or significant reduction of medications in all six treated subjects. However, there was no indication that the problem-solving training with the children added to the effects of the behavioral management classes for parents. There were no noteworthy pre–post differences on the academic measures or the measures of social interaction. On the whole, the authors noted that the children tended to respond in a highly individualized manner. For example, those subjects for whom behavioral management was most effective in controlling behavior at school were not necessarily those who demonstrated the greatest behavioral change at home. Given the length of the problem-solving intervention and the use of behavioral techniques to reward demonstration of new problem-solving skills, it is particularly puzzling that no consistent effects of the intervention were obtained. The small number of children involved certainly qualifies the findings, but the failure of the intervention to produce effects on any of the multiple outcome measures is striking. These findings highlight the individual nature of response to treatment among ADHD children and are consistent with observations of highly individualized outcomes in response to behavioral and pharmacological treatments (see discussions by Pelham et al., in press; Rapport et al., 1988).

When considering treatment outcome research with ADHD children, it is important to examine the impact of cognitive-behavioral training methods relative to and/or in combination with psychostimulant medication treatment. Brown, Wynne, and Medenis (1985) conducted an intervention program similar to that of Douglas et al. (1976) and compared the impact of this program to the effects of psychostimulant medication alone, a combination medication and therapy condition, and a no-treatment control. As assessed at posttest and 3-month follow-up, self-instructional training alone produced significant improvement on only the measures of attention deployment, while medication alone or in combination with cognitive training yielded significant improvement on measures of attention deployment *and* parent and teacher behavior ratings. Neither treatment produced changes on measures of academic achievement. Thus, cognitive training did not yield effects beyond those achieved with psychostimulants. Brown, Border, Wynne, Schleser, and Clingerman (1986) observed that if, in a comparative treatment outcome study, the medication treatment is discontinued prior to posttest, as is the case with the cognitive training, the psychostimulant medication treatment also yields no persisting treatment effects. These findings have the frustrating effect of underscoring both the limitations of the self-instructional methods *and* the urgent need for further development of interventions capable of producing enduring effects.

Results highly similar to those of Brown et al. (1985) were obtained by Abikoff and Gittelman (1985). In addition, Abikoff and Gittelman

(1985) observed that the addition of cognitive training did not facilitate withdrawal from psychostimulant medication for their ADHD subjects. Working with a sample of severely academic-deficient ADHD boys, Abikoff et al. (1988) examined the relative merits of cognitive training plus medication when compared to medication plus remedial tutoring or medication alone. In this study, the cognitive training involved self-instructional training as well as self-monitoring, self-reinforcement, and attack strategy training. Unlike the earlier study by Abikoff and Gittleman (1985), Abikoff et al. (1988) included a behavioral component in which subjects earned points for accurate self-monitoring and experienced response-cost contingencies to encourage accuracy. Results were comparable for all three conditions, suggesting that the self-instructional training did not make a unique contribution to the academic improvement of the children relative to the other treatments examined.

Building on the example of Goodwin and Mahoney's (1975) efforts to train ADHD children to respond more adaptively in a provoking situation, Hinshaw, Henker, and Whalen (1984b) trained small groups of ADHD children via stress inoculation methods (Meichenbaum, 1986). The children were first taught to recognize the physiological cues that signaled the presence of anger and were trained in a variety of cognitive and behavioral strategies for coping with these angry feelings. Children were encouraged to individualize these coping methods and practice their use in a provocative name-calling situation. Control groups were exposed to general principles in social problem solving and perspective taking. Half of the children in each condition received psychostimulant treatment while the other half received placebo. The treatment effects were evaluated by observing each child's response in a behavioral provocation test situation. Compared to their pretreatment response in a similar situation, children in all conditions were more likely to make neutral statements and less likely to laugh, fidget, or display verbal aggression. The children receiving the stress inoculation training received significantly higher ratings on a global measure of self-control and displayed significantly more purposeful coping strategies. Children receiving psychostimulant medication responded less intensely to provocation than did those receiving placebo, but there were no medication-related differences in the content of the children's responses. In the absence of follow-up data or evaluation of the children's responses to other types of provocation it is difficult to know whether any lasting gains were achieved; however, these findings point to the possible efficacy of a carefully focused example of cognitive-behavioral training.

In an investigation exploring the impact of self-evaluation of behavior, Hinshaw, Henker, and Whalen (1984a) trained ADHD children to accurately evaluate the appropriateness of their own social behavior. The self-evaluation group was taught to evaluate their behavior on a simple 5-point scale and could earn reinforcement contingent upon having their self-evaluation match that of an adult observer. The effects of such training on social behavior were examined both with and without concurrent use of psychostimulant medication and were compared to the effects achieved with a traditional external reinforcement system. The findings indicated that the group receiving both self-evaluation training and psychostimulant treatment displayed the most positive behavior, and the self-evaluation-only group was found to be superior to the external reinforcement condition. Other investigators have also observed that self-evaluation or self-monitoring training, both with and without concurrent psychostimulant treatment, can improve the academic and/or social behavior of some children manifesting ADHD and/or other disruptive behavior disorders (Barkley, Copeland, & Sivage, 1980; Chase & Clement, 1985; Neilans & Israel, 1981; Varni & Henker, 1979).

In one of the few published efforts involving the families of ADHD adolescents, Barkley, Guevremont, Anastopoulos, and Fletcher (1992) compared the efficacy of behavioral management training involving parents only, problem-solving and communication training involving parent(s) and child, and structural family therapy involving parent(s) and child. The problem-solving training condition was based on the work of Foster and Robin (1989), which will be discussed further in a later section of this chapter.

When assessed at posttest and 3-month follow-up, all three interventions yielded reductions in reports of negative communication, conflicts and anger during conflict, and improvement in the adolescents' school adjustment. Reductions in adolescents' symptomatology and maternal depression were also noted. Consumer satisfaction with all three treatments was rated as excellent; however, more stringent judgment of clinically significant changes suggested that only 5 to 30% of the families (depending on the criterion used) displayed reliable improvement related to treatment. The authors note that informal reports suggested that families with younger adolescents tended to respond best to the behavioral intervention while those with older adolescents may have been somewhat more responsive to the problem-solving/communication training approach, but the field still has much to learn about effectively matching clients and treatments.

General Conclusions

The results of studies involving children with ADHD behavior suggest that cognitive training can yield evidence of behavioral change with subjects identified as impulsive by task performance measures and with those identified as non-self-controlled by teachers. Even with these less severe populations, however, achieving durable, generalizable change has been difficult. When our consideration turns to children manifesting diagnosed levels of ADHD symptomatology, the outcomes are less encouraging. Nonetheless, there is some promise that cognitive methods may be more effective with ADHD children who are relatively more internal in their locus of control and when training is targeted at improving coping in one or two specific situations. We assert, however, that cognitive treatments are not identical to cognitive-plus-behavioral therapy, and that the latter is more appropriate for the ADHD child.

In their review of cognitive-behavioral methods with this population, Hinshaw and Erhardt (1991) noted that for the child meeting full diagnostic criteria for ADHD, more focused cognitive-behavioral methods such as attribution retraining, anger management training, and self-monitoring/self-evaluation training may have greater value than the more generalized self-instruction or problem-solving training programs. Hinshaw and Erhardt (1991) also noted that to the extent that programs training generalized self-instructions have been effective, even with subclinical populations, they have been *combined with types of behavioral contingencies* that are recognized to be particularly effective with impulsive children (e.g., the use of response-cost contingencies in the work by Kendall and colleagues). In addition, these authors suggest the importance of implementing cognitive-behavioral methods as a means of extending the benefits achieved in the active phase of more traditional operant approaches. For example, training the child to use self-evaluation/self-reinforcement methods as a means of fading an external token reinforcement system.

OUTCOME RESEARCH WITH CONDUCT-DISORDERED CHILDREN

Another group of studies has involved children identified more by their conduct problems than by their impulsivity, inattention, and/or hyperactivity. While the features of these children will be discussed in more detail in Chapter 3, at this point we should note that the primary presenting problems of this population typically involve one or more of the following: (1) various types of noncompliant behavior, (2) defiance of adult authority figures (most commonly parents and teachers), (3) physical aggression with peers or others, and, in more extreme cases (4) serious violations of societal norms and the rights of others. As with ADHD, these studies have involved children manifesting the full range of severity levels, and the treatment protocols that were implemented offer a number of variations of cognitive-behavioral interventions. For the purpose of this review, we examine the results of studies using subjects identified by test data or teacher referral, those identified by parent referral for behavioral problems, and those with subjects who have met clinical criteria for the diagnosis of Conduct Disorder and/or experiencing institutional placement for their difficulties.

Studies with Test- and Teacher-Identified Subjects

While the vast majority of the research in this area has been conducted since 1970, one investigator anticipated the interest in this topic by almost 30 years. Chittenden (1942) designed a training program to help children learn to analyze social situations objectively and select their responses on the basis of this careful analysis. Using a special behavioral situation, Chittenden tested 71 3- to 6-year-olds and selected every child who was in the upper fifth of the sample in dominative initiations or responses and in the lower fifth in cooperative initiations or responses. Children were then matched on age and classroom teacher and assigned to the experimental or control group. Those in the experimental group attended individual sessions in which doll play was used to act out social problem situations. These sessions had three specific aims: (1) to teach the child to discriminate between situations in which satisfactory agreements had been reached and those involving no such agreement; (2) to teach the child ways to work out disagreements in play situations, such as taking turns, common use, or cooperative use; and (3) to make the child aware of successful ways of approaching another child in such play situations. The children were seen daily for approximately 15 minutes over 11 days. The control children were also periodically removed from the classroom to keep the teachers blind to condition assignments. At posttest, the trained children demonstrated significantly less dominant behavior than at pretest. There was also significantly more cooperative behavior in trained subjects at posttest. At 1-month follow-up, however, only the change in dominance persisted. Unfortunately, data on the control group were not presented for comparison with the experimental group. This intervention represents an interesting cross between traditional play therapy techniques and problem-solving training. Despite its early appearance, it incorporates several methodological features, such as age-matched groups, attention controls, and follow-up testing, which, unfortunately, are not always present in more recent studies. The method of subject selection, however, makes it unclear how impaired these children actually were and how many of them were in need of treatment.

Camp and her colleagues (Camp, Blom, Hebert, & van Doorninck, 1977) examined a program designed to teach verbal mediation skills to aggressive second-grade boys. Camp (1977) found that this group of subjects possessed some skills in verbal mediation but failed to use these skills in problematic situations. Accordingly, the treatment involved 30 half-hour sessions that focused on self-instructional training with impersonal tasks and interpersonal problem situations. In addition, training in problem-solving skills was also provided. Twelve treated subjects were compared with 10 who were untreated, and, as another control, Camp et al. (1977) also evaluated 12 "normal" boys selected from the same age group and geographical area. The dependent measures included teacher ratings of aggression and achievement; tests of intellectual ability, achievement, auditory perception, and interpersonal problem solving; and ratings of private speech during testing. At posttest, the treated group showed a significant increase in the teacher ratings of prosocial behavior relative to the control group but no decrease in aggressive behavior. Unfortunately, the teachers were aware of which boys were receiving treatment, so they were not blind raters. The treated subjects showed an increase in the number of solutions provided on the measure of interpersonal problem solving, but these solutions were not of improved quality and frequently included aggressive responses. On the more cognitive measures the treated subjects showed an increase in the number of solutions provided on the measure of interpersonal problem solving, but these solutions were not of improved quality and frequently included aggressive responses. Thus, while the treatment program appeared to have some impact on the children's cognitive functioning, the behavioral effects were much less clear. Other investigators have also reported difficulty in achieving behavioral change with children selected on the basis of their aggressive behavior (Coats, 1979; Dubow, Huesmann, & Eron, 1987; Urbain & Kendall, 1981), but more recent cognitive-behavioral programs have had noteworthy success.

On an encouraging note, Lochman and colleagues have achieved successful outcomes with their Anger Coping Program which was developed for the treatment of aggressive elementary school-aged children (Lochman, Burch, Curry, & Lampron, 1984; Lochman & Curry, 1986). Designed as a school-based group intervention, this program includes discussion and practice of components of effective problem solving, training in the identification of physiological cues of arousal, and practice in the use of appropriate self-talk during provoking situations. Lochman et al. (1984) found that, relative to minimal treatment and no-treatment control conditions, the treated group displayed reductions in aggressive off-task behavior as rated by independent observers, reductions in parent ratings of aggressive behavior, and improved level of self-esteem. These findings have been basically replicated in subsequent research, with the addition of a behavioral goal-setting component producing further improvement (Lochman & Curry, 1986; Lochman, Lampron, Gemmer, Harris, & Wyckoff, 1989).

In some of their investigations, Lochman and colleagues have observed that the aggressive boys who initially had the poorest problem-solving skills were found to make the greatest behavioral improvement after treatment (Lochman, Lampron, Burch, & Curry, 1 985). In a 3-year follow-up of boys treated via the Anger Coping Program, Lochman (1992) reports that treated subjects maintained significant improvement and self-esteem and had markedly lower rates of substance use relative to untreated controls; however, the groups did not differ in their levels of aggressivity or impulsive behavior.

Working with high school students identified as at-risk for dropping out and delinquent behavior, Sarason and Sarason (1981) designed a problem-solving intervention that was presented as a special unit within a regularly required course. The intervention involved 13 class sessions, with the first and last sessions devoted primarily to assessment. The training procedure included the modeling of both the overt behaviors and the cognitive antecedents of adaptive problem solving in both social and cognitive problem situations. These modeled behaviors were then re-hearsed. In one condition subjects viewed live models; in the other treat-ment condition subjects observed videotaped models. A control group received no problem-solving training. At posttest, the treated subjects were able to generate more adaptive alternatives for approaching prob-lematic situations and were able to make more effective self-presentations in a job interview situation than were the controls. In addition, at 1-year follow-up the treated students tended to have fewer absences, less tardi-ness, and fewer referrals for misbehavior. These results are of special interest for they suggest that the intervention was effective at the level of the subjects' cognitive processes and at the level of specific behaviors in real-life problem situations.

Studies with Parent-Identified Behavior Problem Children

Some treatment-outcome researchers studying children with conduct problems have identified their samples based on parental reports of high levels of parent–child conflict and have developed family approaches to the treatment of these conflict-related behaviors. For example, Blechman and colleagues (Blechman, Olson, Schornagel, Halsdorf, & Turner, 1976b; Blechman, Olson, & Hellman, 1976a) examined the impact of a procedure called the Family Contract Game. This technique uses a board-game format to develop problem-solving and contingency contracting skills in families. Component problem-solving skills, such as identifying problems in behavioral terms, gathering relevant information, generating behavioral alternatives, choosing a specific alternative, and evaluating the outcome of the selected alternative, are taught within the game context. After a successful case study application of the game, Blechman et al. (1976b, 1976a) implemented the Family Contract Game with six mother–child dyads. The children (four boys and two girls) ranged in age from 8 to 15 years. The mothers were all employed single parents, ranging in age from 33 to 56 years. These dyads were selected for treatment as a result of parent–child conflict over rules, schoolwork, personal hygiene, and sibling relations. As in Blechman et al. (1976b), unstructured videotaped problem discussions were used as pre–post measures. The intervention was conducted for five 40-minute sessions.

As in the case study, the use of the game procedure resulted in a significant increase in on-task behavior and decreased off-task behavior during problem discussion. This change was apparent in the first intervention session and remained fairly constant throughout treatment. Unfortunately, unlike the case study results, these changes did not persist in posttreatment problem discussions. Decreasing the number of intervention sessions used in the group study versus the case study might be responsible for this failure of generalization. It's also plausible that, given the diverse ages of both children and mothers, the game would need to be modified slightly for use with each particular dyad in order for generalization to occur. These authors should be credited for the extent to which they described their sample of mothers, as well as children, for demographic data on parents are frequently not provided in such studies.

Foster and Robin have also developed an elaborate approach to family problem-solving training (Foster & Robin, 1989; Robin & Foster, 1989). In an initial outcome study, Robin, Kent, O'Leary, Foster, and Prinz (1977) trained 24 mother–child dyads in which the child was 11 to 14 years and who reported experiencing excessive arguing. The treatment was designed to combine the problem-solving model of D'Zurilla and Goldfried (1971) with the communication models of G. W. Piaget (1972) and Gordon (1970). Training emphasized "(1) mutual resolution of disagreements, (2) equalization of decision-making power, and (3) systematic instruction in 'independence-seeking' and 'independence-granting' skills" (Robin et al., 1977, p. 640). Five 1-hour sessions were conducted and session activities included modeling, guided practice, role playing, and social reinforcement of correct problem-solving performance. Pre- and posttreatment assessment included audiotaped discussions of a hypothetical and a real conflict and checklists of home problem-solving and communication skills that were completed by both parents and adolescents. The intervention produced highly significant increases in the use of problem-solving behaviors in the audiotaped discussions of both real and hypothetical conflicts, whereas the control group families showed no positive change or worsened slightly. Specific items on the checklists showed some improvement, but overall the ratings failed to indicate improvement in home problem-solving and communication behaviors. Thus, this intervention appears capable of altering behavior but the altered patterns didn't generalize to real-world settings.

Foster (1979) studied the impact of procedures specifically designed to enhance generalization of these communication and problem-solving skills. Foster's subjects were 28 families complaining of excessive arguing. In this study, both one- and two-parent families were included and the children ranged in age from 10 to 14 years. The treatment groups both utilized the procedures described in Robin et al. (1977); however, one group also experienced procedures believed to enhance generalization, such as homework assignments and weekly discussions of various factors influencing the use of communication and problem-solving skills at home. Training for both groups included seven 1-hour sessions. At posttest, audiotaped discussions indicated a decrease in negative communication in the generalization group, whereas the other treatment and the control group worsened slightly. The problem-solving behaviors coded on these tapes showed no change for any group. Global improvement ratings and self-report ratings of goals, communication targets, and conflict situations showed significantly greater improvement in both treatment groups than in the control group. Also, both treated groups reported use of the skills at home. At 6- to 8-week follow-up, both treatment groups appeared to maintain their treatment gains, with the regular treatment group continuing to improve on some of the measures from posttreatment to follow-up whereas the generalization group worsened slightly on the same measures. These results are somewhat encouraging with respect to the intervention, but the generalization issue remains puzzling. The increased number of sessions for both groups, relative to the Robin et al. (1977) intervention, might have influenced these results, and the use of family-specific measures of change may have resulted in greater sensitivity to treatment effects, but the reason for the nongeneralization group's continued improvement is still unclear.

While past research has clearly demonstrated the efficacy of traditional behavioral child management with behavior problem children, a growing number of studies suggest that adding a problem-solving component to the parent training can enhance child and family outcomes (Dadds, Schwartz, & Sanders, 1987; Griest et al. 1982; Pfiffner, Jouriles, Brown, Etscheidt, & Kelly, 1990). To illustrate, Pfiffner et al. (1990) trained 13 single mothers in behavioral child management. Half of these mothers also received problem-solving training based on D'Zurilla and Goldfried's (1971) problem-solving model (see also D'Zurilla, 1986).

Application of these problem-solving methods was focused on nonchild difficulties such as time management problems, conflicts with ex-spouses, or work-related difficulties. While mothers in both treatment conditions reported significant reductions in child behavior problems at both posttreatment and 4-month follow-up, the addition of the problem-solving component led to greater levels of child improvement at follow-up. Spaccarelli, Cotler, and Penman (1992) reported achieving a somewhat opposite pattern of results, for, in their intervention with the parents of behavior problem children, parents receiving parent training plus problem solving achieved more positive results than those receiving parent training only at posttest, but at 4- to 6-month follow-up both treatment groups appeared to be maintaining similar levels of positive behavioral change. The authors note, however, that significant subject attrition may have biased the results, particularly at the follow-up assessment phase.

Taken together, these studies offer support for the use of family problem-solving training methods when working with children who have been identified by their parents as presenting management problems, and combining problem-solving training with traditional behavioral child management efforts may be particularly beneficial when working with families experiencing numerous life stresses in addition to their child's behavioral difficulties.

Studies with Seriously Conduct-Disordered Samples

This domain of child treatment outcome research can boast of a growing number of studies that evaluate intervention efficacy. The studies to be subsequently reviewed include subjects who meet the criteria for a diagnosis of Conduct Disorder and are in some type of institutional placement and/or experiencing some type of legal system involvement.

As an early example, Sarason (1968) and Sarason and Ganzer (1973) conducted problem-solving training with institutionalized delinquents. In his pilot work, Sarason (1968) reported that a program emphasizing a problem-solving approach to problematic situations via modeling and role playing was effective in producing improved staff ratings of behavior. Sarason and Ganzer (1973) examined the effectiveness of this same program in a more extensive investigation. The subjects were 192 male first offenders ranging in age from 15 to 18 years. Subjects were matched for age, IQ, diagnostic classification, and severity of delinquent behavior and were then randomly assigned to one of two treatments or a no-treatment control condition. The modeling condition, as the authors labeled it, emphasized a practical approach to social problems. The subjects met in groups of four, with two models or tutors per group. The models demonstrated positive and negative approaches to certain problem situations and then the subjects would role-play the same situations. These role plays were taped and played back for discussion. The discussion treatment condition covered the same content as the modeling group but no role play was involved. Both treatment groups met for 16 1-hour sessions over 5 weeks, and within each treatment, half the groups received audiotaped and half videotaped feedback of their group behavior. The results indicated that significantly more subjects in the audiotaped modeling group received favorable case dispositions than all other groups. Those in either the audio- or videotaped modeling groups were significantly more likely to evaluate their institutional experience as positive. Also, modeling subjects were more likely to recall the content and goals of treatment compared to the discussion group (79% vs. 38%) when asked 18 months following treatment. In terms of recidivism, significantly more recidivists were in the control group than were present in either treatment group.

Another successful series of treatment outcome studies has been implemented and reported by Kazdin and colleagues (Kazdin et al., 1989; Kazdin, Esveldt-Dawson, French, & Unis, 1987b; Kazdin, Esveldt-Dawson, French, & Unis, 1987a). Working with 7- to 13-year-olds who were hospitalized on an inpatient psychiatric unit for treatment of their conduct-disordered behavior, Kazdin et al. (1987b) compared the impact of the addition of a 20-session problem-solving skills training program to the conventional hospital program. The problem-solving skills training condition was a combination of the Kendall and Braswell (1985) program (the first edition of this book) and the Spivack and Shure (1974) program. The children receiving the problem-solving training evidenced statistically *and* clinically significant changes on parent and teacher ratings of aggressive behavior that were, in some cases, evident at 1-year follow-up as well as immediately posttreatment.

This treatment was also found to be effective when combined with behavioral child management training (Kazdin et al., 1987a) and when modified to include more opportunities for *in vivo* skills practice (Kazdin et al., 1989). Kolko, Loar, and Sturnick (1990) also report positive outcomes from social cognitive skills training with a sample of inpatient elementary school-aged children meeting criteria for the diagnoses of Conduct Disorder or Conduct Disorder with ADHD. Some positive outcomes with hospitalized aggressive adolescents have also been reported by Feindler, Ecton, Kingsley, and Dubey (1986).

Working with conduct-disordered children in a day hospital program, Kendall, Reber, McLeer, Epps, and Ronan (1990) compared the impact of 20 individual sessions of cognitive-behavioral therapy with the existing hospital treatment in a crossover design, with each treatment phase lasting approximately 4 months. The cognitive-behavioral treatment produced relatively greater changes in teacher ratings of self-control and prosocial behavior and perceived social competence, but no differences were observed on a task performance measure of impulsivity or on teacher ratings of conduct-disordered and hyperactive behavior. Other findings from this study suggested that greater therapist experience providing the cognitive-behavioral therapy was associated with greater positive change in the cognitive-behavioral condition. Though tentative, these data support the idea that the effects of the cognitive-behavioral program are better when experienced cognitive-behavioral therapists provide the treatment program.

Epps, Ronan, and Kendall (1990) reported that subjects who were lower in perceived levels of hostility and aggression and those with more internal attributional styles were more responsive to the cognitive-behavioral therapy provided in Kendall et al. (1990). It should be noted, however, that participation in the cognitive-behavioral treatment seemed to result in those with initially more external attributional styles moving in the direction of increased internality at posttest. Epps et al. (1990) also observed the importance of family factors, with children who perceived their families as having more active parental management evidencing relatively greater improvement.

Other investigators working with seriously disordered samples have opted for greater inclusion of the family in the treatment process. Kifer, Lewis, Green, and Phillips (1974) sought to determine whether negotiation skills could be taught to mother–child dyads simultaneously. Their subjects were two mother–daughter and one mother–son pair in which the children had all had at least one contact with juvenile court. At pre- and posttreatment each pair was observed in the home discussing conflict situations. Also, discussions of simulated conflict situations were recorded prior to and following each session. In both samples of discussions, observers recorded negotiation behaviors (complete communication, identification of issues, suggestion of options) and agreements (compliant vs. negotiated). A multiple-baseline, across-pairs design was used to evaluate the influence of training on the occurrence of negotiation behaviors and agreements. Training followed a model that focused on generating different responses to a given situation, examining the consequences of each response, selecting the desired consequence, and then practicing the chosen response–consequence sequence. Training with each pair continued until the pair displayed two consecutive presession simulated discussions in which all three negotiation behaviors were used between the two pair members. Subjects required from four to six sessions to reach criterion. All three pairs substantially increased their use of negotiation behaviors over baseline levels, but only one pair reached this level of performance prior to being informed of the nature of the termination criterion. In the home observations of real conflict discussions, all pairs showed significant posttreatment increases in negotiation skills and agreements.

This study's use of a termination criterion is an interesting technique, but the failure of two pairs to reach this criterion before being informed of its existence suggests that a motivation to end treatment, as well as improved negotiation skills, may have been responsible for the change. The results also indicated, however, that the negotiation behaviors generalized to home discussions without any explicit generalization training, although the presence of an observer may well have served as a discriminative stimulus for the display of such behavior. The small sample size and the absence of a control group detract from the strength of any conclusions that can be drawn regarding the effectiveness of this intervention.

In an interesting series of studies, Alexander, Parsons, and colleagues (Alexander & Parsons, 1973; Parsons & Alexander, 1973; Klein, Alexander, & Parsons, 1977) worked with delinquent adolescents in a program referred to as functional family therapy. This short-term behavioral intervention focuses attention on contingency contracting but also stresses the modification of family communication patterns with respect to clarity and precision and emphasizes the generation of alternative solutions to family conflicts. Alexander and Parsons (1973) conducted their research with 86 families of delinquents. The children ranged from 13 to 16 years of age and had been arrested or detained for offenses such as running away; shoplifting; habitual truancy; possession of alcohol, soft drugs, or tobacco; or being declared ungovernable. Forty-six families were assigned to the short-term behavioral intervention, 19 participated in a client-centered program, 11 were assigned to a psychodynamically oriented program, and 10 served as no-treatment controls. Treatment effects were assessed via coded videotapes of family interactions and in terms of the recidivism rates of the delinquents. As predicted by the authors, families receiving the short-term behavioral intervention demonstrated significantly more equality of interaction, less silence (more activity), and more interruptions in the videotaped interactions. Recidivism rates were examined during a 6- to 18-month follow-up period. The short-term behavioral, client-centered, psychodynamic, and no-treatment groups obtained recidivism rates of 26%, 47%, 73%, and 50%, respectively. Thus, the short-term behavioral group demonstrated a significantly lower recidivism rate. To study the relationship between the family interaction variables and recidivism, all cases were divided into recidivism and nonrecidivism groups regardless of condition. It was observed that the nonrecidivism group obtained significantly better interaction scores.

Parsons and Alexander (1973) compared the short-term behavioral intervention with a control group using a sample similar to that of Alexander and Parsons (1973). Again, the treatment resulted in significantly improved family interaction. Using an interesting follow-up procedure, Klein et al. (1977) searched for indications of sibling court contact in the 86 families participating in the Alexander and Parsons (1973) intervention. Juvenile court records were examined at a 30- to 42-month interval following the completion of the intervention. The rates of sibling court involvement for the short-term behavioral, client-centered, psychodynamic, and no-treatment groups were 20%, 59%, 63%, and 40%, respectively. These data suggest the positive impact of the short-term behavioral intervention on the family system. In addition to these impressive results by the Alexander research team, positive results with this form of treatment have also been achieved by an independent research group (Gordon & Arbuthnot, 1987).

Working with a sample of 84 serious juvenile offenders and their families, Henggeler, Melton, and Smith (1992) compared the effectiveness of multisystemic treatment with the usual services provided to such offenders. The multisystemic treatment was based primarily on family systems theories of behavioral change, with a recognition of how family difficulties may also be related to peer, school, and neighborhood systemic concerns. In addition, in contrast to some forms of family therapy, the multisystemic approach also emphasized child developmental variables and frequently incorporated cognitive-behavioral therapy based on Kendall and Braswell (1985). The average duration of treatment was 13.4 weeks for the 43 families in the multisystemic condition, with an average of 33 hours of direct contact. Sessions were conducted at the family home or other community-based locations. The control group of serious offenders received court orders involving one or more of the following standard stipulations: (1) curfew, (2) school attendance, and (3) participation in other agencies. Compliance with these stipulations was monitored by each's subject's probation officer in monthly meetings. Results indicated that offenders in the multisystemic program had fewer arrests, fewer self-reported offenses, and, at the 59-week follow-up, had spent an average of 10 fewer weeks incarcerated. Familes in the treatment condition reported increased family cohesion and decreased offender aggression in peer relations. Of particular interest is the finding that these results were *not* moderated by factors such as race, social class, arrest and incarceration history, family relations, or parental symptomatology.

Despite the widespread recognition of how difficult it is to treat seriously conduct-disordered children, this body of research suggests that positive results have been achieved with target samples manifesting clinically significant levels of difficulty. Thus, in contrast to the findings with ADHD children, cognitive-behavioral interventions have a more consistent pattern of significant positive effects and continue to offer greater promise. The programs remediate some of the difficulties of these children and/or offer the families effective coping methods. The demonstration of positive treatment effects with conduct-disordered children is particularly valuable as, unlike ADHD, there are no widely accepted medication treatments that have demonstrated consistent effectiveness with conduct-disordered children who are not also comorbid for ADHD (see Abikoff & Klein, 1992, for discussion of medication use with comorbid children).

Possible explanations for the positive findings with this population of children and adolescents will be discussed in the subsequent section on outcome inconsistency and moderator variables.

OUTCOME RESEARCH WITH LEARNING-DISABLED CHILDREN

As we will discuss in Chapter 3, current thinking about learning disabilities has moved beyond conceptualizations of these difficulties as simply the manifestations of structural anomalies or skills deficits. In some cases, learning disabilities seem more related to problems in the self-regulation of organized, strategic behavior (Harris, 1986a, 1986b). Such children appear to have trouble establishing good correspondence between "saying and doing" in certain academic skill areas. They also seem to struggle to adequately access and then communicate information that is already available to them—either in their text or in their head. It is as though these children impulsively assume they do not know the answer or how to execute a certain attack strategy when the correct answer is not immediately obvious. Many cognitive-behavioral intervention efforts with learning-disabled (LD) children share the general theme of helping these children access and communicate requested information through structured self-questioning or self-guiding statements. We shall describe a few illustrative examples of work in this domain, but we urge the interested reader to seek out additional information in more complete considerations of this topic, such as those by Hughes and Hall (1989), Pressley and Levin (1986), Ryan, Weed, and Short (1986), and Wong et al., (1991).

With reading comprehension, a number of investigators have had notable success in helping LD children implement self-questioning approaches that result in improved comprehension (Graves, 1986; Palinscar & Brown, 1984; Wong & Jones, 1982). For example, Graham (1986; Wong et al., 1991) trained both average and poor fifth- and sixth-grade readers in a self-questioning sequence. Two modes of training were contrasted with a no-treatment control group. In one of the treatment conditions the students were trained in the strategy use via didactic methods, while in the other treatment group the students were trained via self-instructional procedures that were designed to help the students know how to guide and monitor their own use of the strategy. Both treated groups performed better than the no-treatment control on comprehension test results, with the self-instructional group displaying the best performance. Both poor and average readers appeared to improve their skills as a result of the training.

In a slightly different, but equally "cognitive" line of research, Ryan and colleagues (Ledger & Ryan, 1982; Ryan, Ledger, & Robine, 1984) emphasized the value of better cognitive preparation for students to prime them for strategy usage. Their research on informed strategy training suggests that when learners are taught the reasons for the use of a particular strategy and why it may help them, their performance is improved. While outcomes in the field of reading and reading comprehension have been impressive, Wong et al. (1991) note that future research must place more emphasis on helping students clarify the specific nature of their reading comprehension difficulties. This theme is consistent with the growing emphasis placed on training more behaviorally disordered children to be better able to recognize the existence of their social problems and then to enact appropriate strategies.

The use of cognitive-behavioral approaches to remediate written language difficulties is a burgeoning field unto itself, with Harris and Graham making particularly significant contributions to this literature (Graham & Harris, 1989a; Graham & Harris, 1989b; Harris & Graham, 1985, 1988). Drawing on the conclusions of Wong et al. (1991), it appears that the use of self-instructional approaches to improve lower-order skills, such as letter formation, do not yield results that justify the time-intensive use of the procedures; however, the gains resulting from the use of self-instructional methods with higher-order skills, such as composition planning, seem well worth the instructional effort expended. For example, Graham and Harris (1989a) trained fifth- and sixth-grade LD students to generate and organize notes and ideas prior to writing through the use of a series of sequential questions concerning the basic elements of stories (e.g., Who is the main character? Where does the story take place? What does the main character do?) The use of these questions was trained via an eight-step model that included (1) pretraining of any necessary preskills, (2) review of current level of performance and establishment of goals, (3) description of the strategy to be employed, (4) modeling of the strategy and supportive self-instructions, (5) memorization and practice of the strategy steps, (6) supervised practice of strategy steps and self-instruction, (7) independent practice of strategy steps and self-instruction, and (8) discussion and practice of the use of the strategy with other tasks in order to train for maintenance and generalization. Study results indicated that this training significantly improved not only the quality and structure of the students' stories but also their feelings of self-efficacy about writing.

Self-instructional methods have also been implemented with LD students experiencing particular difficulty in mathematics. Successful interventions have included using self-instructions to aid with the acquisition and implementation of the concept of regrouping (Johnston, Whitman, & Johnson, 1980; Keogh, Whitman, & Maxwell, 1988; Whitman & Johnston, 1983), using self-instructions as part of strategy training to help adolescents with two-step word problems (Montague & Bos, 1986), and using cognitive coping interventions to reduce math anxiety in LD children (Kamann, 1989). Various forms of self-instructional training addressing arithmetic difficulties have demonstrated effectiveness with both LD and developmentally delayed students (Leon & Pepe, 1983; Keller & Lloyd, 1989). Research by Barling (1980) emphasized the important role of self-monitoring and self-reinforcement in improving persistence and accuracy on math tasks.

Thus, as the literature on using cognitive-behavioral training to address learning difficulties grows, it yields information that clarifies the value of these methods with various types of learning problems. Generalizing across academic content areas, it appears that cognitive methods are most appropriately used with operations that involve organization and sequencing of certain higher-order processes. When lower-order and/or mechanical processes are involved, such as in the task of learning letter formation, self-instructions may be valuable for a certain brief phase in the learning process but then become unnecessary or even counterproductive once a process or operation has become more automatic.

OUTCOME INCONSISTENCY AND MODERATOR VARIABLES

In almost any review article, the goal is not only to survey the available literature but to attempt to reconcile conflicting findings emerging from different but equally respected research endeavors. Examining the impact of both subject variables and treatment factors is one approach to making sense out of the available treatment outcome results.

Subject Variables

Obviously a number of different features of the child client could have an impact on his/her responsiveness to psychological treatment. Some of these factors, such as child involvement in the session, have been found to be associated with outcome (Braswell, Kendall, Braith, Carey, & Vye, 1985) yet are probably not uniquely relevant to cognitive-behavioral therapy with children. In other words, a high level of child involvement in the session would be expected to be beneficial in virtually any form of child treatment and does not have unique implications for cognitive-behavioral treatment planning. Other types of subject variables, however, might be potentially expected to interact with specific features of cognitive-behavioral interventions and also merit careful attention in treatment planning. A range of different types of subject variables have been examined in relation to cognitive-behavioral treatment, but, at this point, only a few of these variables have amassed data from different investigators that would seem to have real bearing on treatment decision making and outcome. The variables of age/cognitive level, attributional style, and diagnostic/problem status merit special attention.

Age/Cognitive Level

Across investigators, there seems to be increasing recognition that children below the age of 7 or 8 years are generally not good candidates for cognitive-behavioral interventions, at least as these interventions are most commonly implemented. If one is attempting to be consistent with the original Lurian theory guiding the use of self-instructional methods, it must be noted that normally developing children are not hypothesized to have established functional covert self-talk until they are approximately 5 or 6 years of age, so the lack of functional self-talk prior to this point could hardly be defined as a problem. The noted difficulties in replicating the outcomes of Spivack and Shure (1974) or Bornstein and Quevillon (1976) in their work with preschool samples provides further evidence of the potential mismatch between the demands of the cognitive-behavioral methods and the cognitive capacities of preschool children.

Even when considering elementary school-aged children, it is important to consider how age differences might influence the preferred form of training. For example, Bender (1976) found explicit strategy training more effective than a more general type of training with a sample of impulsive first graders, whereas Kendall and Wilcox (1980) and Schleser, Meyers, and Cohen (1981) found conceptual (or more general) training more effective than concrete, task-oriented training with an *older* group of children (non-self-controlled 8- to 12-year-olds). Taken together, more studies involving adolescent clients seemed to achieve positive outcomes than was observed with other age groups. In their meta-analysis of self-instructional training research, Dush, Hirt, and Schroeder (1989) also observed a relatively more positive impact in studies involving adolescent samples. Including problem-solving training with the parents of behaviorally disordered children, in addition to traditional child behavioral management training, also appears to add to the potential efficacy of such treatment (Pffifner et al., 1990).

Kendall (1977) emphasized the importance of considering the cognitive level of the child when designing a cognitive-behavioral intervention program. This is not to say that such training would not be reasonable and effective with retarded or learning-disabled children, because there are examples of its effectiveness with such populations (e.g., Guralnick, 1976; Wagner, 1975). Cognitive capacity or level seems to operate much like the age factor, with children at a lower stage of cognitive development requiring more task-specific and concrete training and brighter children responding best to more abstract training. Research by Cohen et al. (1982) found that cognitive level, as assessed from a Piagetian stage perspective, interacts with type of training in predicting outcome, thus underscoring the role of level of cognitive development. Based on anecdotal accounts from our own work, trainers working with borderline retarded children found it effective to increase the amount of tutor modeling in each session and to apply the self-instructional steps to sports or games that the subjects already knew how to play. With these alterations of the program, the less intellectually developed children mastered the self-instructional approach to problems by the sixth or seventh session, although the average-range children typically master the steps by the third or fourth session.

Thus, it seems extremely important for the tutor to work at the child's pace, not the experimenter's, if the ultimate goal is the child's mastery of the material. The format utilized in most experimental intervention programs is, however, more concerned with controlling for amount of training time than with achieving a prespecified degree of content/skills mastery. While this is understandable from a design standpoint, such an approach allows little opportunity for attention to the individual learning rate or style of the child. Clinical applications can and should be sensitive to the learning needs of the individual client.

Attributional Style/Locus of Control

Kopel and Arkowitz (1975) noted that a child's feeling of personal control over his/her life might influence his/her responsiveness to any type of self-control intervention. One's beliefs or expectations about control over events has been assessed via the concepts of locus of control and attributional style. Locus of control (Rotter, 1966) refers to a generalized tendency to expect that events are controlled by either factors internal to one's self (e.g., ability or effort) or factors external to one's self (e.g., luck or powerful others). Attributional style refers to a tendency to explain or perceive the cause of events that have occurred as the result of factors that may be internal or external to oneself, that may be stable or changeable over time, and/or that may be highly situationally specific or more generalized. The possible role of these factors was first examined with respect to self-instructional training by Bugental et al. (1977). As previously described, attributional and medication status were found to interact with treatment approach (self-instructional training vs. social reinforcement) on a task performance measure of impulsivity at posttest but not at 6-month follow-up. In addition, self-instructional training produced more durable increases in perceived control than did the social reinforcement condition, but the latter condition produced longer-lasting improvement in teacher ratings of hyperactivity (Bugental et al., 1978).

The finding that those high in personal control improved more with self-instructional training is consistent with the work of Schallow (1975), who found that undergraduates high in internal orientation, as measured by Rotter's Locus of Control scale (Rotter, 1966), were more successful in self-modification of a number of behaviors. Braswell, Koehler, and Kendall (1985) reported that children who tended to attribute positive behavioral change to effort also tended to obtain positive change on teacher ratings of classroom behavior. Correspondingly, attributing positive behavioral change to luck was negatively associated with change on teacher ratings. Epps et al. (1990) have observed that, among a sample of conduct-disordered children participating in a day treatment program, the presence of a more internal attributional style was related to greater change with cognitive-behavioral treatment. Consistent with the observations of Bugental et al. (1978), Epps et al. (1990) also reported that children initially rating themselves as more external in their attributional style at pretreatment were rating themselves as relatively more internal at post-treatment.

In a study that speaks even more directly to the issue of changing a child's attributional status, Reid and Borkowski (1987) contrasted traditional self-instructional training with self-instructional training that also included specific coaching of the children to make effort attributions regarding their successes and mistakes, with successful task performance being attributed to good effort at using the self-instructional strategies and mistakes attributed to failure to use the strategies. Relative to the traditional training and control conditions, the self-instructions plus attribution retraining group displayed a more reflective cognitive style and an increased sense of personal causality. In addition, at 10-month follow-up, a hyperactive subsample displayed more positive teacher ratings of social behavior.

Thus, while attributional style may mediate one's initial response to cognitive-behavioral treatment, such treatment can also function as a means of changing the extent to which one perceives events as being caused by factors internal or external to one's self.

Diagnostic/Problem Status

Within the category of disruptive behavior disorders, it appears that the type of primary difficulty manifested by the child influences the probability of positive outcome following cognitive-behavioral treatment. As clearly indicated in the preceding discussion of specific research, while cognitive-behavioral efforts have value for mild to moderately impulsive children, particularly when implemented with appropriate contingencies to support learning, they are not always of value, at least as most commonly implemented, for alleviating other primary symptoms of children manifesting clinically significant ADHD behavior. In a very interesting and puzzling contrast, there is a significant body of research to support the view that cognitive-behavioral interventions can achieve meaningful change with children displaying clinically significant levels of aggression and oppositionality, but relatively less support for the use of these methods with more mildly conduct-disordered children (Abikoff & Klein, 1992). This conclusion is different from that drawn in the first edition of this book and is the result of more recently emerging negative findings with samples manifesting ADHD behavior and positive findings with samples displaying more conduct-disordered symptomatology. Two possible reasons for this observation come to mind. One explanation concerns the structure of the intervention and will be discussed in the subsequent section on treatment factors, but the other relates to features of the subject or, perhaps more accurately, represents a subject by treatment content interaction.

As will be discussed in the next chapter, hypotheses about the cognitive mechanisms that lead to observed symptoms have been offered concerning both ADHD and conduct-disordered behavior. It is possible that at least some of those mechanisms hypothesized to be involved in the sequence that leads to conduct-disordered behavior are more amenable to change via psychosocial therapeutic methods than may be the case with the mechanisms leading to the expression of the primary symptoms of ADHD. For example, the processing issues or lapses thought to be involved in inattentive behavior seem to occur over very brief spans of time, perhaps milliseconds, that do not easily allow the interposition of new cognitive coping techniques. In contrast, in the problematic interactions displayed by conduct-disordered children, certain perceptual biases may be enacted quickly yet the ensuing social interactions usually involve some degree of reciprocal exchange that plays out over several seconds or even minutes. Thus, even if the conduct-disordered child's first thought was to respond with some expression of hostility, there might be a few moments in which he/she could reconsider the wisdom of this response and enact some type of well-trained cognitive coping tool to deescalate the situation (e.g., consideration of alternative interpretations of the situation, consideration of the consequences of inappropriate behavior, use of calming self-talk or other relaxation methods). Thus, helping conduct-disordered children, and possibly those who are both ADHD and conduct disordered, "stop and think" could result in a reduction of inappropriate responses—at least in certain situations in which interactions occur over a matter of seconds and minutes rather than milliseconds. This view is consistent with the findings of successful use of cognitive-behavioral methods with conduct-disordered samples *and* with ADHD samples when the specific issue being addressed was coping with anger-producing situations rather than coping with inattention and impulsivity in a more generalized context. In line with this reasoning, while it may be difficult to prevent the ADHD child's initial attentional lapse, which occurs quickly, one could theoretically train the child to recognize the occurrence of such a lapse and to use this observation as a signal to redirect one's self to the task at hand (assuming adequate motivation for task completion, which may not always be the case unless supplemental incentives have been provided). This possibility is consistent with the positive results reported in using self-monitoring/self-evaluation methods to improve both the on-task and social behavior of ADHD children.

The success of cognitive-behavioral approaches with a variety of learning difficulties also suggests a good match between features of the expression of the underlying deficit and the time requirements of enacting the selected coping mechanisms. Clearly, the value of this speculation awaits a better understanding of the underlying cognitive/biological mechanisms associated with all the disruptive behavior disorders and learning difficulties. But even with our current knowledge base it still seems logical to ask ourselves whether the behavioral issue being targeted actually plays out in a manner that allows time for second (and, it is hoped, more constructive) thoughts to occur. If not, it may not be realistic to pursue attempts to train these second thoughts.

Treatment Factors

Features of both the structure and content of the various interventions reviewed could certainly help explain variations in reported outcome.

Family/Parental Involvement

As discussed by Braswell (1991), different forms of cognitive-behavioral intervention vary greatly in terms of the degree and formality of family and/or parental involvement in treatment. Many self-instructional training programs did not include parents or, at best, informed parents of procedures but required no documentation of actual use of the methods by the parents. In contrast, many problem-solving training programs directly intervened with parents and child together. Considering both studies involving parent-identified behavior problem children and those with more severely conduct-disordered children, there appears to be a tendency for these family interventions to more commonly report positive outcomes; in fact, with regard to the literature just reviewed one could conclude that it is the use of cognitive-behavioral therapy with children alone that should be questioned, not the use of cognitive-behavioral approaches with parents and families.

This family involvement issue may also be related to the observed differences in outcomes between ADHD and conduct-disordered samples of children. With the exception of the Barkley et al. (1992) work with ADHD adolescents and their families, none of the cognitive-behavioral interventions with ADHD children had a high degree of structured parental involvement, including documentation of attempts to use trained skills in the home environment. In contrast, several of the successful cognitive-behavioral interventions with more conduct-disordered samples target the child and parent rather than the child alone. It should also be noted that although the outcomes achieved in the Barkley et al. study were not as robust as those observed with some of the conduct-disordered samples, positive findings did emerge from all three family-oriented intervention conditions.

Braswell and Bloomquist (1991) have proposed that greater, more structured parental involvement in the training process, as well as coordinated home–school use of problem-solving methods could lead to greater efficacy of cognitive-behavioral approaches with ADHD samples. Along with Gerald August, Braswell and Bloomquist are currently conducting a large-scale evaluation of this home–school intervention model. Thus, the real impact of such an approach remains to be seen. In addition, several of the successful efforts with conduct-disordered samples did not have a formal parental component, so family involvement is clearly not the only issue determining the success or failure of a given program.

Individual versus Group Intervention

Studies conducting both individual and group training in self-instructional procedures have achieved some positive results, but only the Kendall and Zupan (1981) study specifically contrasted these two modes of training. Although the results indicated that relatively comparable change was achieved by both individual and group training, the "group" condition may not have maximized its potential. That is, children in the group training "took turns" as opposed to engaging each other in the use of stop-and-think self-talk. There seems to be a geater tendency to use group methods among the interventions developed from a problem-solving perspective relative to those evolving from a self-instructional training perspective, and given the merging of these perspectives in recent efforts, there has also been an increased use of groups. Given that the presence of other children, particularly children inclined to have difficulties, one would hypothesize that the group format provides a training context more similar to the social context in which trained skills are to be used. Procedures described in Chapter 7 provide more group opportunities for practice and learning of the cognitive skills.

Training Targets

The most common focus of problem-solving training was teaching children to generate behavioral alternatives to problem situations. Several interventions (Giebink, Stover, & Fahl, 1968; Sarason & Sarason, 1981; Spivack & Shure, 1974; Shure & Spivack, 1978) explicitly assessed this skill at pre- and posttreatment, and all three studies reported increased generation of alternatives following treatment. Spivack and Shure took the next step of ascertaining whether the individual children improving in generation of alternatives were also demonstrating behavioral improvements. These authors found that children improving in generation of alternatives were also more likely to be rated as behaviorally adjusted following treatment.

The interventions conducted with parent–child pairs tended to emphasize communication and negotiation skills in addition to problem-solving techniques. Alexander and Parsons (1973) conducted an analysis similar to that of Spivack and Shure by assessing whether those parent–child dyads which demonstrated improved communication skills were actually the families with lower recidivism rates. Their findings did indicate a significant relationship between better skills and lower rates of recidivism. On the other hand, Foster (1979) reported that one of her treatment groups displayed slightly worse communication skills at posttest, yet this group showed the most long-lasting improvement on self-report measures of the family's specific goals, communication targets, and conflict situations. Thus, in some cases, the role of the skills emphasized in training remains unclear.

One could also reformulate the earlier discussion concerning differences in the cognitive mechanism of ADHD versus conduct-disordered children as being an issue of training targets. For example, interventions that explicitly targeted anger coping skills, particularly anger cue recognition and rehearsal of specific coping strategies in response to these cues, seemed to achieve more positive outcomes, whether conducted with ADHD or conduct-disordered samples (Hinshaw, Henker, & Whalen, 1984b; Lochman & Curry, 1986).

Use of Explicit Behavioral Contingencies

Despite being considered exmples of cognitive-behavioral therapy, many of the interventions previously discussed did not actually include any form of explicit behavioral contingency, or, in some cases, contingencies were not well integrated into the program to truly serve the role of fostering learning and appropriate in-session behavior. For example, Douglas et al. (1976) invoked contingencies only when children were extremely unmanageable, and Abikoff and Gittelman (1985) provided only social praise and noncontingent reinforcement (Kendall & Reber, 1987). Brown et al. (1985) and Brown et al. (1986) used no formal contingencies. As previously noted, perhaps one reason for the positive results achieved in the research by Kendall and colleagues has been the inclusion of carefully chosen contingencies that match the needs of the training sample. In the case of the current program, the use of response-cost contingencies seems ideal for addressing the impulsive behavior so characteristic of the targeted sample. The use of explicit behavioral contingencies has been relatively less common in past problem-solving training efforts, but several of the more successful programs have included behavioral contingencies to support learning and change (e.g., Lochman et al., 1984). The research is incomplete, but it is our opinion that behavioral procedures (e.g., proper modeling, contingencies) are a valuable facet of any program designed to teach interpersonal problem-solving skills.

Self-Reinforcement

In addition to the use of externally managed contingencies, some interventions incorporate a self-reinforcement component. Many of the self-instructional approaches and interventions deriving from an operant formulation of self-control include self-reinforcement as a routine element of the trained sequence. Nelson and Birkimer (1978) specifically contrasted the effects of self-instructional training with and without self-reinforcement and reported that self-instructions with self-reinforcement produced improvement on the MFF, whereas self-instructions alone did not. The general findings of the more operant self-regulation studies discussed previously also suggest that self-instructions are most effective in achieving behavioral change when the treatment package includes a self-reinforcement component. These interventions, however, also included self-monitoring and self-evaluation activities, so the specific effects of self-instructions versus self-reinforcement remain unclear. One might conceptualize the self-reinforcement component as providing a specific goal toward which the child can direct his/her behavior. When self-instructions are taught as a means of achieving this goal, they may be more effective than if presented in a more ambiguous or "goal-less" framework in which the advantage of using the self-instructions is not obvious to the child.

CONCLUSIONS

The present review leads us to conclude that cognitive-behavioral interventions have achieved outcomes that justify their use in certain situations and/or with certain target populations. ADHD children would appear to benefit from self-monitoring/self-evaluation training and may benefit from anger/frustration management training and attribution retraining focused on increasing their sense of control over the events they experience. Currently, it appears that individual, child-focused training in general self-instructional methods (without contingent behavioral programming) does not produce meaningful and enduring change in ADHD children. With conduct-disordered, oppositional children (some with and without ADHD) both child-focused and family-oriented training seem capable of producing positive change.

Learning difficulties that involve higher-order capacities and problems in the organization of thought also seem responsive to cognitive-behavioral intervention while those related to lower-order or mechanical skills issues may not be well suited for such intervention approaches.

Compared to the status of the literature at the time of the publication of the first edition, it appears that we now have more information to guide both clinical decision making and future research pursuits. As previously discussed, there is an urgent need to better understand the cognitive/biological underpinnings of the targeted difficulties, so that intervention efforts can be increasingly refined and the field can become more realistic about the types of issues that are responsive to and appropriate for psychotherapeutic intervention.

CHAPTER 3

Nature of the Deficit: The Target Sample for the Treatment

t is our position that the outcomes of treatments are optimal to the degree that they focus on the exact nature of the specific deficit troubling the identified youth. We advocate that treatments not be prescribed according to the therapists' theoretical allegiances or professional affiliations but, rather, that the deficit shown by the child and, more specifically, the exact features associated with the deficit, should determine the type and manner of treatment that is provided. No one intervention strategy or philosophy can be optimal for all of the various types of childhood disorders.

The cognitive-behavioral procedures detailed in this book were developed for use with children manifesting impulsivity and deficits in self-control. Children falling into this group are often described as impulsive, attention disordered, overactive, disobedient to adult authorities, externalizing or undercontrolled (Achenbach, 1966; Achenbach & Edelbrock, 1978), and/or aggressive toward others. They may carry psychiatric diagnoses such as Attention-Deficit Hyperactivity Disorder (ADHD), Oppositional Defiant Disorder (ODD), or Conduct Disorder. Children experiencing learning problems or formal learning disabilities may also exhibit impulsivity. Still other children may not meet formal criteria for a particular diagnostic grouping but nonetheless may struggle with issues related to impulsivity.

Describing the target group is not difficult, but certain complexities are present. For instance, while the intervention described herein has its main historical antecedents within behavioral attempts to enhance self-management of discrete behaviors, the recipients of the intervention have frequently been described in terms of the traditional psychiatric labels or labels more associated with trait or temperament theories (Buss & Plomin, 1975; Chess, Thomas, & Birch, 1968) than with behavioral formulations. In our description of the target population and the nature of its deficits, we are comfortable with a blending of perspectives, but our comfort rests on certain assumptions. We recognize that certain patterns of behavior that may be reflective of problems in self-management (e.g., blurting out in class, inability to sit still, difficulties in effective attention deployment) are also symptoms of some psychiatric syndromes. We acknowledge that some diagnostic labels are accompanied by assumptions regarding etiology and prognosis that are not accepted by some cognitivists and/or behaviorists. Current thought regarding the disruptive behavior disorders, however, suggests that these syndromes may be the final common manifestations of a wide range of etiological agents. Thus, using a diagnostic label does not imply acceptance of a specific theory of causation.

On the other hand, we also agree that "prior to systematic assessments, there is no reason for interpreting certain clinical disorders (such as hyperactivity, antisocial or criminal behavior, depression, or academic failure) as being self-management disorders by definition" (Karoly, 1981, pp. 92–93). Using one of Karoly's examples, a child's antisocial behavior, such as vandalism, may not be the result of an inability to manage or control his/her behavior but rather the result of a conscious decision to imitate a peer or adult model, even while cognizant of the potential long-term consequences. Thus, while most children diagnosed with ADHD can be assumed to manifest some degree of impulsivity, the presence of a self-control problem should be established, not assumed, for ODD and Conduct Disorder. Even with ADHD children, one must determine whether the child's impulsivity is severe enough to merit being the focus of intervention.

In the remainder of this chapter, we discuss important features of disruptive behavior disorders and learning disabilities. Given the emphasis placed on impulsivity, however, we first provide an overview of this construct.

IMPULSIVITY

The significant research attention that has been directed toward defining and understanding impulsivity is, in large part, the result of the seminal work of Jerome Kagan and his colleagues (Kagan, 1965, 1966; Kagan, Rosman, Day, Albert, & Phillips , 1964). In a fascinating series of studies on children's problem-solving abilities, Kagan et al. (1964) were struck with the stability of a child's tendency to adopt a reflective or impulsive approach to solving problems that required the analysis of several simultaneously available response alternatives. These investigators introduced the term *conceptual tempo* to refer to this dimension of reflective versus impulsive responding. The impact of a child's conceptual tempo was hypothesized to be greatest when the child was confronted with a moderate degree of response uncertainty. In other words, a child's tendency to be impulsive versus reflective would not necessarily be apparent in problem situations in which the child knew the right answer immediately or had no idea of the correct response. Rather, this tendency would be observable when the child perceived the right answer as being present but felt somewhat uncertain about which response it might be. These early studies introduced the MFF test as a means of identifying a child's conceptual tempo. This original line of research found that children identified as cognitively impulsive were more likely to make errors on reading tests and tests of serial learning. Cognitively impulsive boys were also observed to be more distractible and overactive relative to reflective boys.

Kagan et al. (1964) postulated that at least three factors might contribute to a child's development of an impulsive versus reflective style. First, constitutional/biological factors were implicated, particularly prenatal and perinatal experiences but also hereditary influences. Second, the child's degree of involvement with the task was felt to impact processing style. Children with high performance standards would be more likely to be reflective since they cared about the quality of the produced response, while children who did not care about the quality of their answer would be less likely to reflect. Third, the child's degree of anxiety about his/her ability to perform the task could also influence conceptual tempo. Kagan et al. (1964) speculated that children anxious about their ability to perform adequately might have difficulty tolerating the silence or delay necessary for accuracy on a task like the MFF and, as a result, would answer too quickly in an attempt to appear competent. Unfortunately, such unreflective responding is more likely to yield an inaccurate response and further increase the child's anxiety.

With its emphasis on biological factors, motivational factors, and the role of coexisting emotions/beliefs activated by the task, Kagan's explanation for the display of impulsivity in a particular situation is highly consistent with more recent formulations concerning the behavior of ADHD children (see Barkley, 1990; Braswell & Bloomquist, 1991). Readers aware of the history of cognitive-behavioral constructs may also find it interesting to note how Kagan's notion about the potential impact of anxiety upon competent task performance foreshadows Bandura's (1977) later discussion of the concept of self-efficacy beliefs and their impact on performance.

In the decades since Kagan's original research was introduced, the concept of impulsivity has been scrutinized intensely. On one hand, there has been increasing recognition that impulsivity is probably not a unitary construct (Block et al., 1974). Kendall and Wilcox (1979) pointed out the need to recognize signs of impulsivity at both a cognitive or executive level and a behavioral level. The cognitive level is consistent with Kagan et al.'s (1964) view of impulsivity as an inability to adequately evaluate an array of alternative problem solutions. Behavioral impulsivity, however, concerns the inability to inhibit unwanted verbal or physical acts. This elaboration of the construct has been important in helping the field acknowledge the complexity of impulsivity, but elaboration has also led to definitional confusion.

As discussed by Milich and Kramer (1984), impulsivity has been defined in the research literature in increasingly diverse ways, including such views as an inability to delay gratification; an inability to stop, look, and listen; an inability to inhibit motor movements; and poor planning ability. Clearly, such definitional diversity has made it difficult to compare findings across studies and has slowed the development of an organized body of research concerning this construct.

Even if one holds to defining cognitive impulsivity via performance on the MFF test, the relationship between this form of cognitive impulsivity and other cognitive and behavioral dimensions is unclear. Like the original Kagan studies, some more recent investigators have observed an association between MFF-defined cognitive impulsivity and a host of other variables, including increased errors on other types of information processing tasks, increased presence of soft neurological signs, and elevated levels of platelet monoamine oxidase (MAO) activity (Stoff et al., 1989; Vitiello, Stoff, Atkins, & Mahoney, 1990; Walczyk & Hall, 1989). Other researchers, however, have not been able to demonstrate a relationship between MFF-defined cognitive impulsivity and other task performance measures of impulsivity, much less global ratings of behavior (Day & Peters, 1989; Gaddis & Martin, 1989; Milich & Kramer, 1984).

And what are the implications of this confusing state of affairs for the psychologist attempting to understand and treat a reportedly impulsive child? First, if the child is referred for treatment by virtue of his/her alleged impulsivity, the clinician must carefully delineate the nature of this impulsivity. The reader is referred to Chapter 4 ("Assessment Issues and Procedures") for further discussion of how to accomplish this goal. Second, the clinician must be sensitive to other aspects of the cognitive, affective, and behavioral pattern presented by the child. In this regard, the remaining sections of this chapter provide information about conditions commonly associated with impulsivity. Third, we hope at least some of our readers will be inspired to begin or continue research efforts aimed at clarifying the connections among and between cognitive impulsivity, behavioral impulsivity, and other types of behavioral disinhibition.

Conditions Associated with Impulsivity

Difficulties involving impulsive behavior appear to be extremely common in both clinical and nonclinical samples of school-aged children and adolescents. Conners (1980) estimated that 60% to 70% of the clients at child guidance clinics are referred by parents or teachers because the child's externalizing behavior has made him/her a management problem.

Based on teacher ratings of nonclinical samples of school-aged children, Werry and Quay (1971) report that 30% of males and 13% of females were described as overactive, 46% of males and 22% of females were rated as disruptive, 43% of males and 25% of females were said to have a short attention span, and 26% of males and 11% of females were rated as disobedient and difficult to discipline. Learning difficulties that may involve impulsivity are also relatively common.

In this section we present an overview of the diagnostic conditions most commonly associated with impulsivity, including ADHD, ODD, Conduct Disorder, and learning disabilities. These diagnostic labels and their descriptions are based on criteria from the revised third edition of the *Diagnostic and Statistical Manual of Mental Disorders* (DSM-III-R) (American Psychiatric Association [APA], 1987), as these are the standards in effect at the time of the publication of this book. The development of DSM-IV (APA, 1991) is, however, well under way, with publication expected in 1994 or 5. Where relevant, we make note of issues and questions concerning the DSM-III-R criteria that may be addressed in DSM-IV.

In addition, there are certainly children who appear to struggle with impulsivity in certain specific contexts who do not otherwise qualify for any formal diagnostic category. For example, some children become mildly anxious and behave impulsively when faced with a multiple-choice exam but do not display more generalized signs of distress. Other children may be impulsive in social contexts yet not display impairment in other areas of functioning. Given the success reported in cognitive-behavioral outcome studies with nonclinical populations (as discussed in Chapter 2), one could expect that these children would be favorably responsive to the intervention methods described in this volume.

ATTENTION-DEFICIT HYPERACTIVITY DISORDER

ADHD is the disorder most readily associated with problems of impulsivity. As noted in the first chapter, impulsivity is one of the criteria of ADHD, so, by definition, virtually all children with ADHD manifest some impulsive behavior. In DSM-III-R, the label Undifferentiated Attention-Deficit Disorder is used to refer to those children manifesting marked attentional difficulties in the absence of other symptoms of ADHD.

Prevalence

Estimates of the prevalence of this condition vary with the number of raters involved and/or the stringency of the identification criteria employed by a particular investigator, with most estimates falling in the range of 3 to 5% of the population of school-aged children (Barkley, 1990). Target samples defined only by teacher ratings tend to produce higher estimates of prevalence, usually on the order of 5 to 15% of an elementary school-aged sample (Huessy, 1974; Trites, 1979). Studies involving trained mental health professionals or multiple raters produce estimates in the range of 1 to 6% (Lambert, Sandoval, & Sassone, 1977; Rapoport, Quinn, Burg, & Bartley, 1979).

Sex Ratio

All investigators have observed higher prevalence rates among males, with ratios varying from 3:1 to 9:1 (Barkley, 1990). Experienced clinicians and educators report that attentional difficulties without hyperactivity may occur more equally in boys and girls, but this observation awaits empirical confirmation. Generally speaking, ADHD girls have not received the intense research attention afforded ADHD boys, so firm conclusions cannot be drawn about sex differences in a number of aspects of symptom expression.

Behavioral Pattern

The key symptoms displayed by ADHD children involve various manifestations of attentional difficulties, impulsivity, and, in many cases, hyperactivity. It is expected that there will be some changes in the formal diagnostic criteria for this condition in DSM-IV, but current DSM-III-R criteria require that the child display at least 8 of the following 14 symptoms:

1. Often fidgets with hands or feet or squirms in seat;
2. Has difficulty remaining seated when required to do so;
3. Is easily distracted by extraneous stimuli;
4. Has difficulty awaiting turn in games or group situations;
5. Often blurts out answers to questions before they have been completed;
6. Has difficulty following through on instructions from others;
7. Has difficulty sustaining attention in tasks or play activities;
8. Often shifts from one uncompleted activity to another;
9. Has difficulty playing quietly;
10. Often talks excessively;
11. Often interrupts or intrudes on others (e.g., butts into other children's games);
12. Often *does not seem* to listen to what is being said to him/her;

13. Often loses things necessary for tasks or activities at school or at home; and
14. Often engages in physically dangerous activities without considering possible consequences (APA, 1987).

These symptoms must have emerged before age seven and have been observed for at least 6 months. In addition, it is emphasized that the child's symptoms must be judged in terms of his/her mental age. Thus, if an 8-year-old's cognitive functioning is at the level of a 6-year-old, his/her behavior must be evaluated in terms of what would be considered appropriate for a 6-year-old.

In DSM-IV, there is a possibility that children will be required to display features from two or three symptom groupings (i.e., either inattention and hyperactivity/impulsivity or inattention, impulsivity, and hyperactivity), depending on data emerging from field trials with the criteria. It also appears that the DSM-III-R diagnosis of Attention-Deficit Disorder (ADD) without hyperactivity will be reinstated, perhaps with more formal recognition of the daydreaming and low energy/apathy that seem to accompany this condition. It is acknowledged that there is still controversy about whether ADD with and without hyperactivity represent variants of the same disorder or are two relatively unrelated conditions (APA Task Force on DSM-IV, 1991).

Despite changes in labels and the relative emphasis given to certain symptoms, there is high agreement that the attentional difficulties of ADHD are manifested as distractibility, inability to listen, difficulty concentrating and completing projects, and difficulty sticking with play activities. These problems are more likely to be displayed in situations that require greater self-application, such as the classroom, and DSM-IV criteria may in fact require that symptoms be present in a structured setting (e.g., school or occupation). Attentional difficulties may not be observed when the child is in a novel or one-to-one work situation.

As previously discussed, ADHD is also notable for impulsivity, which may be displayed via a wide range of behaviors, including impulsively responding on psychoeducational tasks, verbally blurting out and interrupting, and physically irritating others. Impulsiveness is also manifested as a tendency to shift excessively from one activity to another and an inability to await one's turn in a group or game situation. In some situations impulsiveness may be tantamount to recklessness. For example, ADHD children may run into the street or climb dangerous structures, not because they are necessarily thrill seeking but because they do not pause to reflect on the potential danger of their acts.

While attentional difficulties are now considered the primary symptom of ADHD, hyperactive behavior is often the most obvious symptom manifested by some ADHD children. This overactivity is typically manifested by intense and undirected energy, fidgetiness, inability to sit still, and, in some cases, a reduced need for sleep (Cantwell, 1977). In the classroom this overactivity often takes the form of running, jumping, remaining out of seat without permission, and restlessly moving arms and legs even when seated (Cammann & Miehlke, 1989; Luk, 1985). In an observation of 26 hyperactive preschool children and 26 controls, Schleifer et al. (1975) rated behavior that occurred during periods of free play and structured play. No differences were observed between the hyperactives and controls in the free-play situation, but in the structured-play situation hyperactives exhibited significantly higher rates of "up" and "away" behaviors. Weiss (1975) also has difficulty distinguishing hyperactives from normals in a free-play situation. Jacob, O'Leary, and Rosenblad (1978) observed hyperactives and normals in both open and traditional classrooms. The hyperactive children displayed the same activity levels in both settings, but normals were less active in the more structured, traditional settings. In light of these findings, it seems that the overactivity of these children becomes problematic because of their inability to modulate or manage their activity level in accordance with the demands of their environment rather than simply because of the absolute amount of activity they display.

Secondary Problems

In addition to the major symptoms of ADHD, investigators have increasingly recognized the socially inappropriate nature of the child's behavior and the deficits in self-control implied by such behavior (Barkley, 1982, 1990; Routh, 1980). Both ADHD children with and without noteworthy levels of hyperactivity seem to be at increased risk to experience peer rejection (Carlson, Lahey, Frame, Walker, & Hynd, 1987). Such children appear to be as likely to blurt out inappropriate statements to peers as they are to blurt out in classroom situations. For example, when observed in play groups, ADHD children can emit 3 times as many aggressive behaviors and 10 times as many negative verbal statements as peers (Pelham & Bender, 1982).

Other factors that frequently accompany ADHD symptoms include poor school achievement and specific learning disabilities. Mendelson, Johnson, and Stewart (1971) found that 58% of the hyperactive children in their sample had failed one or more grades in school by the time they reached adolescence. Poor school performance has been observed by many other investigators (Hechtman, Weiss, Finkelstein, Werner, & Benn, 1976; Minde et al., 1971; Weiss, Minde, Werry, Douglas, & Nemeth, 1971), and it is particularly surprising when many ADHD children are known to score at or above the average range on individually administered IQ tests. While some school difficulties appear to be the direct result of the child's primary ADHD symptom, these children are also at elevated risk for a formal learning disability. Reading disabilities, speech and language difficulties, and other written language problems seem to be particularly common among ADHD children (Braswell & Bloomquist, 1991), but the exact percentage of overlap between ADHD and formal learning disabilities depends greatly on the particular definition of learning disabilities being used (Barkley, 1990).

Conduct problems, including physical and verbal aggression, have also been observed more frequently in children and adolescents exhibiting ADHD symptoms than in controls (Abikoff, Gittelman-Klein, & Klein, 1977; Safer & Allen, 1976; Szatmari, Offord, & Boyle, 1989). The overlap of ADHD and Conduct Disorder has led some investigators to question whether the two entities can be viewed independently (Prior & Sanson, 1986). While recognizing that comorbidity may be the rule rather than the exception among the disruptive behavior disorders, the current weight of scientific opinion favors the recognition of separate categories of attentional difficulties/hyperactivity and serious conduct problems (Abikoff & Klein, 1992; Hinshaw, 1987; Lahey, Stempniak, Robinson, & Tyroler, 1978; Milich, Loney, & Landau, 1982; Roberts, Milich, Loney, & Caputo, 1981).

Developmental Shifts

Several authors have pointed out the importance of recognizing developmental shifts in symptomatology (Barkley, 1990; Cantwell, 1977; Denhoff, 1973; Ross & Ross, 1976; Wender, 1971). The mothers of children who were later diagnosed as hyperactive often report that these children were particularly demanding and irritable infants who tended to be irregular in their physiological functioning (Ross & Ross, 1976). Using Sanders's (1962) five levels of adaptation, hyperactive children and their mothers appear more vulnerable to difficulties in establishing regular patterns (Ross & Ross, 1976). It should be noted, however, that these disturbances are not characteristic of hyperactive, acting-out children alone (Thomas, Chess, & Birch, 1968).

During the preschool years, the symptoms of overactivity, attentional difficulties, and low frustration tolerance may appear. In addition, these children may continue to exhibit irregularity of mood and physiological functioning. These children may also seem to have no sense of danger and to be unaffected by disciplinary efforts that are successful with other children (Cantwell, 1977). As mentioned previously, Schleifer et al. (1975) did observe differences of certain off-task behaviors in preschool children in structured but not free-play situations. Again, it must be cautioned that single symptoms such as overactivity are relatively common at this age, and not all of those preschoolers who appear somewhat overactive go on to manifest the full symptoms of ADHD (Weiss, 1975); in fact, Campbell (1990) noted that the majority of children descibed as inattentive at 3 or 4 years of age are also described as being significantly improved within 3 to 6 months. There is, however, a subgroup of young, extremely active children who are already displaying a symptom pattern that will continue throughout later stages of development (Weiss & Hechtman, 1986).

During the early elementary school years, the behaviors noted previously persist and may become much more noticeable. Given the demands of the classroom environment, children who had not previously exhibited problems of attention or activity level may begin to have such difficulties at school. As mentioned earlier, many of these children develop academic problems. These academic and behavioral difficulties may feed into the development of both poor self-concept and poor peer relations.

Ross and Ross (1976) suggested that adolescence may represent a more difficult time for the child than the primary school years, for even though activity level may decrease, the attentional, educational, and social difficulties persist and antisocial behavior may appear. One follow-up study of adolescents originally diagnosed as ADHD in elementary school found that approximately 20% of the original sample exhibited normalized behavior by adolescence. The remaining 80% continued to manifest some degree of behavioral or cognitive–developmental abnormality, with 43% continuing to require active treatment (Lambert, Hartsough, Sassone, & Sandoval, 1987). These findings are particularly interesting, because the original sample was derived from a community screening effort rather than from clinic referrals, with community-based screening less likely to produce a sample that would be biased toward negative long-term outcomes. The outcomes were, however, much like those reported with samples originally derived from clinical settings (Weiss & Hechtman, 1986). In a follow-up of a sample of rigorously diagnosed ADHD subjects, Barkley and colleagues found that over 80% continued to meet criteria for the disorder when assessed as adolescents (Barkley, Fischer, Edelbrock, & Smallish, 1990; Fischer, Barkley, Edelbrock, & Smallish, 1990). Thus, in samples selected for manifesting a noteworthy level of disturbance, there is a high degree of continuity of difficulty into adolescence.

Cognitive Deficits

Many investigators have written about the cognitive or mediational deficits that are believed to be responsible for the observed difficulties of ADHD children. The work of Douglas and her colleagues has been central to the identification of possible defective processes (Douglas &

Peters, 1979). As reviewed by Douglas (1983), processes under consideration include "(1) the investment, organization, and maintenance of attention and effort; (2) the inhibition of impulsive responding; (3) the modulation of arousal levels to meet situational demands; (4) an unusually strong inclination to seek immediate reinforcement" (p. 280). Douglas notes that any of these processes could play a dominant role in producing the observed behavioral difficulties or these processes could be interacting in a complex manner.

Considering research on attention processes, Douglas (1980) observed that hyperactives do no worse than normals on paired association tasks involving pairs that are meaningfully associated or, in other words, pairs that provided a "built-in" strategy for remembering. On the other hand, the performance of hyperactives is notably worse when the pairs involve arbitrary associates that require the subject to generate his/her own strategy for remembering. This observation has been replicated by subsequent research (August, 1987; Borcherding et al., 1988). In a review of studies examining the task strategies of impulsive and reflective children, Cameron (1977) reports that the majority of the studies found impulsives less likely to display focusing strategies. In his own research, Cameron found impulsives more likely to approach the task in a disorganized manner and make guesses or attend too narrowly to a particular stimulus dimension, rather than systematically utilizing strategies that would rule out competing alternatives. Interestingly, Cameron also observed that even when impulsives were able to verbalize more effective task approaches, they seemed to have difficulty maintaining attention to their own task rule and would make choices inconsistent with their verbalized strategy. Tant (1978) compared the performance of matched groups of hyperactive, reading-disabled, and normal controls on matrix solution tasks. The hyperactive children were distinguishable from both the other groups, for they appeared to conduct less thorough perceptual analyses of the arrays and displayed a lack of information about what constituted "efficient" questioning. These findings are particularly interesting since the three groups were matched for verbal IQ and an effort was made to help all subjects remain highly motivated.

These findings dovetail nicely with theories about metacognitive development and self-regulation. Brown (1975) and, much earlier, Vygotsky (1962) distinguished between knowledge that is acquired in a non-self-conscious, relatively automatic way and knowledge that must be consciously, deliberately sought. This difference may be relevant for understanding the cognitive strengths and weaknesses of non-self-controlled, hyperactive children. For instance, Brown (1975) has suggested that successful performance, at least in most Western cultures, demands the application of deliberate, systematic learning strategies, particularly given the fact that most exercises within formal education are likely to appear contrived and serve no obvious purpose from the child's perspective— leaving little chance of spontaneous learning. The normally developing child displays gradual, stepwise movement toward greater concious control over his/her own learning (Vygotsky, 1978) and an accompanying increase in the ability to self-monitor and self-evaluate his/her problem-solving efforts (Brown, 1987). Unfortunately, the ADHD child seems to face increasing difficulty as learning tasks require greater levels of conscious self-regulation and organization, with the majority of these children experiencing academic difficulties throughout their school career (Hoy, Weiss, Minde, & Cohen, 1978; Mendelson et al., 1971; Minde et al., 1971; Weiss et al., 1971). These perspectives are consistent with the notion of cognitive deficiencies associated with lack of behavioral control (Kendall & MacDonald, in press).

In a contrasting view, Barkley (1990) has recommended a shift from conceptualizations that explain ADHD as a disorder of attention to a view of ADHD as a neurologically based insensitivity to consequences. This lack of responsiveness to consequences is believed to account for the ADHD child's observed difficulties with following rules or guidelines, particularly in situations in which consequences are delayed, weak, or not present. Barkley asserts that, relative to an attention-focused perspective, this viewpoint more adequately addresses the extent to which observed symptoms seem to be the product of a child-by-environmental interaction, not just the result of features of the child. In addition, this conceptualization is consistent with emerging biological findings concerning decreased activity in brain reward centers and findings regarding the role of dopamine pathways in regulating motor behavior and instrumental learning (Barkley, 1990).

Ultimately, a clear understanding of the underlying deficits of ADHD children must await clarification of potential causal factors, as will be discussed in the following section. Regardless of the mediating deficits, however, cognitive-behavioral interventions offer the capacity to intervene at both the level of cognitive strategy development with the child and at the level of implementing problem-solving approaches with the child and his parents and teachers in order to enhance the salience of particular consequences for appropriate and inappropriate behaviors.

Causal Hypotheses

Everything from prenatal trauma to sugar consumption to parenting style has been postulated as a possible cause for ADHD behaviors (see reviews by Barkley, 1990; Braswell & Bloomquist, 1991). Some current scientific evidence favors the role of a biological factor, particularly malfunctioning in the processing of certain neurochemical transmitters that seem to result in underactivity in specific brain regions associated with the regulation and planning of behavior and overactivity in regions involving the experiencing of sensorimotor stimulation. It is unclear the extent to which this malfunctioning could be the result of genetic factors or pre-, peri-, or postnatal trauma. While these emerging biological explanations may be applicable to large numbers of ADHD children, for certain individuals, specific bioenvironmental processes, such as maternal consumption of alcohol during pregnancy, may also play a role in producing attentional difficulties. For other subgroups of ADHD children, factors such as lead poisoning, specific food or inhalant allergies, or extremely unstructured environments of rearing may also be involved.

Given this confusing state of affairs, most investigators endorse the viewpoint of Hartsough and Lambert (1982, 1984, 1985), who argue that "both individual differences in the organic and psychological make-up of the child and individual differences in the family and social environment contribute to whether or not a child is identified as hyperactive" (p. 273). The general trend in the field toward biological explanations will likely promote related research. Nevertheless, the balanced multicausal perspective of Hartsough and Lambert may transcend any one particular trend in the field.

Prognosis

It was once held that ADHD remitted at puberty (Bakwin & Bakwin, 1966; Bradley, 1957; Laufer & Denhoff, 1957). Subsequent research suggests that while overactivity does generally decrease for some ADHD children between the ages of 12 and 16, many of the associated problems persist.

Studies of long-term outcomes for ADHD children have struggled with a number of serious methodological problems, including subject attrition or dropout, the failure to include control groups of other types of psychiatrically impaired children, and the use of subject identification measures that confound ADHD with ODD and Conduct Disorder.

Despite these numerous flaws, the conclusions of various studies have been quite consistent in suggesting that while a substantial minority of subjects do not continue to display symptoms into adolescence, the majority of subjects do evidence persisting symptomatology. Adolescents with persisting ADHD symptoms are at risk to develop more antisocial spectrum behaviors but are not at elevated risk for other disorders. Some early reports on long-term outcome suggested that ADHD children were at risk to develop criminal behavior as adults. Later research has indicated that the risk for criminal behavior is largely mediated by the development of serious conduct-disordered behavior in adolescence or early adulthood. ADHD adolescents without Conduct Disorder are, nevertheless, at risk for academic difficulties. Treatment with psychostimulant medication alone has not been found to reduce the risk for negative behavioral outcomes in adolescence, but multimodal intervention, involving medication plus individual, family, and educational intervention, has been found to reduce the risk for the development of more serious delinquent behavior (Barkley, 1990; Braswell & Bloomquist, 1991).

OPPOSITIONAL DEFIANT DISORDER AND CONDUCT DISORDER

Children who meet the diagnostic criteria for either ODD or Conduct Disorder represent a second group that commonly manifests problems stemming from impulsivity. Unlike ADHD, however, impulsivity is not, by definition, part of the symptom picture of the ODD or conduct-disordered child. From a societal perspective, these children clearly display poor judgment, but the presence of impulsivity issues must be assessed rather than assumed.

Prevalence

Conduct difficulties that could result in a diagnosis of either ODD or Conduct Disorder are the most frequently occurring form of childhood behavioral problem in both samples of children derived from clinics and those drawn from the general population (McMahon & Wells, 1989). As noted with ADHD children, the rate of occurrence of single symptoms associated with ODD and Conduct Disorder is extremely high; in fact, at certain ages the display of select antisocial behaviors seems to be the rule rather than the exception. For example, early longitudinal/developmental studies have found that as many as 53% of 6-year-old boys engage in lying but by 12 years the percentage has dropped to 10% (MacFarlane, Allen, & Honzik, 1954). Among teenagers, as many as 60% admit to engaging in at least one form of conduct-disordered behavior, such as drug abuse, physical aggression, vandalism, or arson (see discussion by Kazdin, 1987). Of course, the use of the formal diagnostic labels such as ODD or Conduct Disorder requires that a constellation of symptoms be present. When formal criteria are applied, prevalence estimates range from 3 to 9% of the population of children under age 18 (APA, 1987; Rutter, Cox, Tupling, Berger, & Yule, 1975; Trites, Dugas, Lynch, & Ferguson, 1979).

Sex Ratio

As discussed by McMahon and Wells (1989), whatever the age or sample studied, boys are referred for treatment of conduct problems, are diagnosed as conduct disordered, and admit to the display of antisocial behavior more frequently than do girls, with sex ratios varying from 4:1 to 12:1 (Kazdin, 1987; McMahon & Wells, 1989). The occurrence of ODD is believed to be more common in boys prior to puberty but equally common in postpubertal members of both sexes (APA, 1987).

Behavioral Pattern

It is anticipated that DSM-IV will result in some changes in the criteria for ODD and Conduct Disorder. These changes are most likely to relate to the expressed nature of the relationship between ODD and Conduct Disorder. If the standards established in DSM-III-R persist, ODD and Conduct Disorder will continue as two separate categories, with the clear acknowledgement that ODD typically precedes the development of Conduct Disorder, but not all children manifesting ODD go on to display Conduct Disorder. An alternative, however, might involve the creation of a new diagnosis, Disruptive Behavior Disorder, that would include ODD and Conduct Disorder. This new category would include three severity levels: level 1 for Oppositional Defiant Type (which basically matches the DSM-II-R ODD diagnosis), level 2 for Moderate Conduct Type (which includes the less severe symptoms of the current Conduct Disorder diagnosis), and level 3 for Severe Conduct Type (which includes the most serious symptoms from the current Conduct Disorder criteria) (APA, 1991).

According to DSM-III-R, children displaying persistent difficulties with losing their temper, arguing with and defying adults, deliberately antagonizing others, and blaming others for their difficulties are most accurately diagnosed as manifesting ODD. If the child's behavior escalates into violations of societal norms and the basic rights of others, as illustrated by behaviors such as stealing, destruction of property, and physical violence, the diagnosis becomes Conduct Disorder. Most children diagnosed as conduct disordered may have previously met criteria for a diagnosis of ODD.

The DSM-III-R standards also specify three types of Conduct Disorder behavior. The group type describes those who primarily commit antisocial acts as part of a peer group activity. The solitary aggressive type presents with a primary symptom of physical aggression, which does *not* occur in the context of peer group activities. Finally, the undifferentiated type refers to those who present with a mixture of symptoms that cannot be classified in either of the two preceding groups. At the current time, it is unclear which Conduct Disorder subtypes will be retained in DSM-IV, and it is hoped that the diagnostic field trials will yield data that will help with this determination.

As previously noted, many of the specific symptoms of ODD and, to a lesser extent, Conduct Disorder may be manifested by normally developing children, but it is possible to clarify the significance of the observed behavior by evaluating it in terms of several dimensions. As described by Kazdin (1987), the extent to which the child's behavior is *repetitive* and *chronic* helps sort out the degree to which a clinically significant problem may exist. Also, the *range* or *breadth* of antisocial behaviors displayed provides a clue to the seriousness of the condition. Finally, the presence of low-frequency but *high-intensity behaviors*, such as setting fires or assault with a weapon, indicates that the child's conduct problems are well beyond normal variations in age-appropriate behavior.

Secondary Problems

As noted with ADHD, the conduct-disordered or ODD child often displays serious secondary or comorbid difficulties. The overlap between ADHD and ODD/Conduct Disorder is quite high (Hinshaw, 1987; Reeves, Werry, Elkind, & Zametkin, 1987). Some investigators have suggested that hyperactivity may be a necessary ingredient for the display of severe Conduct Disorder (Loeber, 1985) and studies of long-term prognosis clearly indicate that the outcome for children displaying both disorders is worse than for children displaying either difficulty alone (Hinshaw, 1987).

Children with ODD and Conduct Disorder are also at risk for academic difficulties. The presence of a reading disability in conduct-disordered children has been a particularly common finding (Rutter, Tizard, Yule, Graham, & Whitmore, 1976; Sturge, 1982), and the conduct-disordered child is much more likely to have been held back a grade in elementary and junior high school (McMahon & Forehand, 1988). While some of the observed academic difficulties might be the direct result of Conduct Disorder symptoms such as truancy, recently emerging data also suggest that underachievement is associated with the presence of coexisting ADHD (Frick et al., 1991).

An association between Conduct Disorder, ODD, and depression has also been noted (Chiles, Miller, & Cox, 1980; Jensen, Burke, & Garfinkel, 1988). While Curry and Craighead (1990) have noted that depression in a conduct-disordered child or adolescent may have different features or correlates than depression in those without serious social maladjustment, the recognition of depressive features in the ODD or conduct-disordered child may still have important implications for adequate treatment planning.

Finally, by definition ODD and conduct-disordered children tend to have interpersonal conflicts with their parents and other adults in the community. Both observational and sociometric data indicate that these interpersonal difficulties extend to peer relations, with conduct-disordered children more likely to be aversive with other children and, not surprisingly, to experience rejection from their classmates (Kazdin, 1987; McMahon & Forehand, 1988).

Developmental Shifts

Most diagnostic formulations of ODD and Conduct Disorder assume that the child first manifests symptoms of ODD in the home. Over time, the display of these symptoms may spread to other environments and the degree to which the rights of others are violated may increase, thus resulting in a diagnosis of Conduct Disorder. As previously noted, if the child also displays symptoms associated with ADHD, such as inattention, impulsivity, and overactivity, this seems to increase the probability of the persistence of severe difficulty. If the symptoms of Conduct Disorder continue past age 18, the person is then diagnosed as manifesting Antisocial Personality Disorder.

Several investigators have proposed models for the developmental progression of Conduct Disorder behavior (Edelbrock, 1985; Loeber, 1989; Patterson & Bank, 1989). Interestingly, all three of these viewpoints emphasize the central role of noncompliant behavior and the parental response to this behavior as the gateway to other forms of difficulty. Selected examples of these viewpoints will be discussed in a subsequent section on the role of the family.

Cognitive Deficits and Distortions

The issue of cognitive or mediational deficits and distortions in children with ODD and Conduct Disorder has not received the same level of research attention afforded ADHD children, but there is a growing body of literature exploring possible cognitive dysfunctions (Kendall & Mac-Donald, in press) that may play a role in producing ODD or Conduct Disorder symptomatology. In particular, research has focused on social cognitive problem-solving skills that are believed to mediate overt social behavior. The work of Dodge on the social information processing of aggressive children deserves special mention.

In an interesting series of studies, Dodge and colleagues have demonstrated that aggressive children attend to fewer cues when attempting to understand the meaning of others' behavior (Dodge & Newman, 1981) and are more likely to encode and recall cues with hostile connotations than are nonaggressive children (Dodge, Pettit, McClaskey, & Brown, 1986). Dodge (1980) observed that aggressive boys were significantly more likely to infer that a character presented in a hypothetical provocation acted with hostile rather than benign or neutral intent. Other lines of research on the problem-solving abilities of aggressive children suggest that they generate fewer and more aggressive solutions to social dilemmas than do comparison children (Asarnow & Callan, 1985; Richard & Dodge, 1982), and they may have deficits in both means–end thinking and perspective-taking ability (Asarnow & Callan, 1985; Gurucharri, Phelps, & Selman, 1984). The reader is referred to Feindler (1991), Kendall, Ronan, and Epps (1990), and Lochman et al. (1991) for further discussion of the cognitive characteristics of conduct-disordered children.

Causal Hypotheses

ODD and Conduct Disorder may be the result of a variety of biological and environmental factors. Data from both twin and adoption studies suggest the role of genetic factors but also indicate that certain features of the environment interact with genetic predisposition to moderate or increase risk. The specific mechanism through which genetic factors exert an influence is not clear. Some investigators, such as Mednick (1975), have suggested that arousal patterns of the autonomic nervous system may be inherited and these patterns influence the extent to which the child will learn to refrain from inappropriate behavior in an effort to reduce fear and arousal (Kazdin, 1987). A number of environmental influences have also been delineated. In particular, the role of parent–child interactions has emerged as significant, with some parents of conduct-disordered children unintentionally promoting antisocial behaviors through their own misdirected parenting efforts. Other environmental factors such as parental marital discord, parental psychiatric disturbance, overcrowding in the home, and characteristics of the school setting may increase a child's risk for the development of conduct-disordered behavior.

Prognosis

The presence of ODD symptoms clearly constitutes a risk for the emergence of Conduct Disorder, and, in turn, the persistence of symptoms of Conduct Disorder into late adolescence puts the individual at risk for the development of Antisocial Personality Disorder. Loeber (1982) noted that those who have an early onset (before age 10), who display different types of disordered behavior, who act out frequently, and who do so in more than one setting are the most likely to manifest continuing difficulties. In addition to being at risk for criminality and Antisocial Personality Disorder, such individuals are at high risk for substance abuse and dependence, lowered educational achievement, poor occupational adjustment, higher rates of medical and psychiatric hospitalization, and widespread interpersonal difficulties (Kazdin, 1987).

LEARNING DISABILITIES

Some children identified as learning disabled (LD) may display impulsive behavior that is appropriate for treatment via cognitive-behavioral approaches. Even more than was the case with ODD and Conduct Disorder, however, the presence of impulsivity in an LD child must be established through careful assessment rather than assumed. The term *learning disability* covers an extremely broad category of difficulties. Presenting symptoms may range from problems with specific academic skills to general behavioral traits, such as poorly organized study behaviors or speech and language disturbances. This state of affairs has led Taylor (1988) to note that "the only characteristic shared by all children with learning disabilities is that they do not perform in school in accordance with expections" (p. 402).

A number of different definitions of learning disability have been offered (see discussions by Myers & Hammil, 1990; Taylor, 1988; Westman, 1990), but the definition with the greatest pragmatic impact is that contained in Public Law No. 94-142. This law provides LD children in the United States with a legal guarantee to special educational services. This definition emphasizes the presence of a severe discrepancy between achievement and perceived ability level and age in one or more of the following areas: basic reading skill, reading comprehension, written expression, oral expression, listening comprehension, mathematics calculation, or mathematical reasoning. To qualify as a learning disability, the severe discrepancy cannot be the result of other factors, such as mental retardation, emotional disturbance, or limited educational opportunity. Interestingly, after much debate over the extent to which ADHD children are eligible for learning disabilities services, the U.S. Department of Education has issued a letter of clarification in which it states that ADHD was intended as a condition to be covered by Public Law No. 94-142 (U.S. Department of Education [USDE], 1991).

We hope the information presented in this section will be helpful to the reader, but given the complex, multifaceted nature of learning disabilities, we urge all interested parties to obtain additional information from a variety of texts and review chapters on this topic (see Hooper &

Willis, 1989; Myers & Hammil, 1990; Silver & Hagin, 1990; Taylor, 1988; Swanson, 1991; Westman, 1990).

Prevalence

A report from the USDE (1988) indicated that during the 1986–1987 school year, 4.8% of public school children between the ages of 3 and 21 received some level of learning disabilities programming. Speech and language services were provided to another 2.85%. Given the variable nature of the screening and referral process for receiving special educational services, it is commonly assumed that there are more children who have some form of learning disability than there are children receiving learning disabilities services. Most screening surveys have produced estimates indicating that 5 to 15% of school-aged children have some type of learning disability (Myers & Hammil, 1990; Taylor, 1988).

Sex Ratio

As with the previously discussed disorders, boys are more likely to be identified and to receive services for learning disability, ratios ranging from 2:1 to 5:1 (Taylor, 1988). In particular, boys seem at elevated risk for difficulties with reading and written language skills.

Behavioral Pattern and Cognitive Deficits

Unlike ADHD and ODD/Conduct Disorder, learning disability cannot be discussed in terms of a few key symptoms, for both the child who can read but not make progress in math and the child with solid math skills but poor reading could be labeled learning disabled. Rather, one must discuss the major subgroups within the broad category of learning disability and consider possible subtypes within each subgroup. The existence of many forms of learning disability has logically led to the development of a number of different methods of classification.

As discussed by Hooper and Willis (1989) and Taylor (1988), some significant subtyping systems emphasize identifying specific neurocognitive skills deficits, such as perceptual–motor difficulties, immediate verbal memory deficits, or sequential processing problems. Other systems rely more on grouping children in terms of the particular academic domain that appears to be difficult for them. For example, Myers and Hammil (1990) described learning disabilities as falling into the categories of disorders of spoken language, disorders of written language (reading, writing, spelling), disorders of arithmetic, and disorders of reasoning. Obviously, the particular system in use will determine both the behavioral pattern and the cognitive deficits observed in a specific sample of LD children.

Cognitive-behavioral researchers have shown a steadily increasing interest in understanding the cognitive deficits of LD children. While many current definitions assume the presence of structural or abilities deficits, some emerging research suggests that even if such deficits do exist, the child's poor academic performance may also be the result of difficulties in the self-regulation of organized learning strategies. Investigations of the LD child's tendency to use less helpful self-talk, his/her failure to produce metacognitive task strategies without prompting, and the manifestation of maladaptive attributions all point to a potential match between the needs of the LD child and the issues targeted by cognitive-behavioral interventions (Wong et al., 1991).

Secondary Problems

In addition to variations in the behavioral pattern manifested by LD children, a number of potential secondary difficulties have been observed.

As previously discussed, a significant subgroup of ADHD children also meet formal criteria for being labeled learning disabled, with comorbidity more common in samples derived from clinical rather than community surveys (Ackerman & Dykman, 1990). Barkley (1990) noted that the exact percentage of overlap between the two conditions is highly dependent on the particular definition of learning disability being employed. Definitions focusing on IQ–achievement discrepancies tend to produce higher estimates of learning disability in ADHD samples, while those based on achievement cutoff scores tend to yield lower rates. While attentional difficulties are one of the hallmarks of ADHD, LD children have been observed to perform more poorly than normals on measures of sustained attention (Krupski, 1986). LD children are also considered to be at elevated risk for both motor and perceptual–motor difficulties, such as poor left–right orientation (Myers & Hammil, 1990). In addition, low self-esteem and feelings of demoralization have been identified as common secondary difficulties for LD children (Porter & Rourke, 1985).

Developmental Shifts

The child's developmental status appears to impact the recognition, manifestation, and severity of learning disabilities. Clearly, it is difficult to detect certain kinds of learning disabilities in preschoolers, such as problems with mathematics, because we do not expect children to be able to master certain concepts until they are older. Other types of difficulties, however, such as problems with speech and language functioning, can be recognized at an early age and early intervention is encouraged.

Swanson (1991) has suggested that in light of the developmental nature of the learning process, learning disabilities probably may be manifested in different ways at different ages. For example, a child who has difficulty with automization and memorization of information might first appear to have difficulties with reading but not math, for early math concepts do not require the same degree of involvement with the problematic processes as is the case with early reading skills. By the time the child is expected to master multiplication tables, however, he/she may begin to experience serious math difficulties due to the demand for automatization and memorization of multiplication facts. While Taylor (1988) notes there is little data on this topic, it is widely believed that learning disabilities become more common and more severe in advancing grades due to both the cumulative impact of failure to master basic skills and processes and the more advanced problem-solving demands placed on children at higher grade levels.

Causal Hypotheses

As with much of human behavior, there is mounting evidence to suggest that learning disabilities may be the result of a combination of both constitutional and social/environmental factors.

As summarized by Taylor (1988), whereas much of the evidence is indirect, it appears reasonable to assert the existence of biological antecedents for some forms of learning disability. Central nervous system irregularities have been demonstrated through computerized EEGs and autopsy examination, with many of these irregularities seeming to be the possible result of a variety of pre- and perinatal difficulties involving inadequate oxygen to the brain. In addition, some specific forms of learning disability, such as reading disability, may have a genetic basis (Myers & Hammil, 1990). Although representing a small subset of all LD children, there are clearly some students who manifest learning difficulties as a direct result of definitive, continuing neurological disorder (e.g., epilepsy, head injury, cerebral palsy) and chronic medical conditions (e.g., asthma, diabetes, endocrine disorders) (Taylor, 1988).

Other investigators, however, point out that data from large epidemiological studies suggest that at least perinatal distress has proved to be less important than socioeconomic factors in predicting later school difficulties (Westman, 1990). Being born into an advantaged sociocultural environment appears to help constitutionally vulnerable children compensate for possible deficits, while those born into disadvantaged environments may be at risk to develop learning disabilities regardless of their constitutional risk status (Taylor, 1988). Some formal definitions of learning disability exclude those children whose difficulties can be accounted for by limited educational opportunities. There is, however, no question that the learning of many children is directly impacted by environmental factors such as insufficient early experiences, cultural/linguistic differences, malnutrition, and/or poor teaching (Myers & Hammil, 1990).

Prognosis

Most experts agree that the prognosis for LD children is extremely variable. While such children are at high risk for continuing difficulty with academic skills, other factors may influence the degree to which the child continues to be at risk for social–emotional difficulties and problems with occupational adjustment. As discussed by Taylor (1988), the child's emotional status could be highly influenced by his/her own motivation and coping skills as well as the degree of acceptance by parents and teachers. Occupational status may be more influenced by the student's original economic status than by the presence of learning disability. Taylor (1988) notes that other potentially significant factors include the initial severity of the learning difficulty, the child's age when the difficulty was recognized, the specific versus generalized nature of the problem, the child's other cognitive abilities, and his/her responsiveness to intervention efforts.

ROLE OF THE FAMILY

Whatever the childhood issue being examined, it is important to consider the impact of the child's social/emotional context. For the developing child, no social/emotional context is more important than his/her family environment. As discussed by Braswell (1991), parents play a crucial role in defining the child's issues as a "problem." Factors such as the parent's understanding of normal development, the parent's own emotional state, and the parent's degree of involvement in the child's difficulty may influence the extent to which the child's behavior is considered problematic. In addition to their role in defining the child's behavior as problematic, parents are often directly implicated in causing, maintaining, or moderating the expression of the behaviors in question.

From a developmental perspective, Kopp (1982) has noted that even though parental or caregiver factors probably do not play a direct causal role in the development of capacities for self-regulation, these factors may play an important facilitative role. That is, there is nothing that parents do or fail to do that is directly responsible for their child's displaying developmentally appropriate self-regulation, but their actions may enhance or interfere with the natural unfolding of these skills. For example, Lytton

(1976) reported that parents' use of language and general approach to caregiving related to their 2-year-old's compliance skills, and the work of Golden, Montane, and Bridger (1977) suggested that parental expectations and use of verbal techniques were influential factors in determining the child's ability to delay his/her behavior in a laboratory task. Kopp (1982) also noted that stressful family events may be associated with changes in demonstrated level of control. Using divorce as an example, Kopp (1982) found that when newly divorced mothers lowered their demands for their child's independence and provided less communication and reasoning, child control was impaired. This suggests that family stress is sometimes translated into parental behaviors that have the ultimate effect of reducing the child's demonstrated level of self-control. These findings are interesting in that they identify a possible pathway or mediating link between family stress and child misbehavior. The potential complexity of these pathways has been further demonstrated by the observation that the impact of stress upon parenting behavior may interact with other factors, such as the sex of the child. For example, Jouriles, Pfiffner, and O'Leary (1988) observed that mothers in conflicted marital relationships were less likely to punish deviant behavior in girls and more likely to direct disapproval statements to boys.

Understanding the impact of stress on family functioning is also of particular relevance because it is widely observed that the families of children with disruptive behavior disorders have unusually high rates of a variety of stress-producing factors. Disrupted marriages and interpersonal conflict have been reported to occur at higher than average frequencies among the parents of delinquents or children with conduct disorders (Glueck & Glueck, 1950; Johnson & Lobitz, 1974; McCord, McCord, & Gudeman, 1960; Nye, 1958; Rutter, 1974). Interestingly, despite the high degree of overlap between ADHD and Conduct Disorder, one of the more reliable distinctions between the two groups involves lower rates of social adversity and parental psychopathology in the families of ADHD children relative to the families of ADHD plus Conduct Disorder and Conduct Disorder–only samples (Biederman, Munir, & Knee, 1987; Lahey et al., 1988; Schachar & Wachsmuth, 1990).

In a more fine-grained analysis, Paternite, Loney, and Langhorne (1976) examined the relationship between parenting variables, socioeconomic status (SES), and both primary and secondary symptoms associated with hyperactivity. Inattention, fidgetiness, hyperactivity, judgment deficits, negative affect, and incoordination were considered primary symptoms; aggressive interpersonal behavior, control deficits, and self-esteem deficits were labeled secondary symptoms. While boys from low-SES families demonstrated higher rates of secondary symptoms, the parenting variables were found to be even stronger predictors of these symptoms. Thus, the parents' caregiving style was more strongly associated with the presence of aggression, impaired self-control, and low self-esteem than was the family's SES. Interestingly, neither parenting variables nor SES was consistently associated with the presence of primary symptoms, suggesting that family variables are implicated in the expression of some, but not all, of the class of externalizing behaviors.

Family factors also appear to play a role in exacerbating or moderating the impact of a learning disability upon the child. As summarized by Taylor (1989), attributional research suggests that children are negatively impacted when their parents have low expectations for them and when the parents have a tendency to attribute any positive outcomes to luck or the actions of others. Also, counterproductive child management practices, lack of encouragement for the child, and limited parental attitudes toward learning can seriously impair the child's learning and school functioning.

Family factors have also been associated with response to treatment and general prognosis. Several investigators have reported a positive relationship between quality of parental management and favorable short-term response to stimulant treatment for hyperactivity (Conrad & Insel, 1967; Loney, Comly, & Simon, 1975). With respect to more long-term outcomes; it has frequently been observed that family disturbance and parental abnormalities were associated with more antisocial child outcomes (Mendelson et al., 1971; Minde et al., 1971, 1972; Weiss et al., 1971). Child acceptance by the parents also seems to moderate some of the more negative emotional outcomes for LD and ADHD children (Ziegler & Holden, 1988).

Of course, while parental factors may affect the expression of certain behaviors by the child, there is clearly a reciprocal relationship between the actions of virtually all parents and children. As Barkley (1981) stated, "Parent and child behaviors can be viewed as a reciprocal feedback system where the behavior of each serves as both controlling stimuli and consequating events for the behavior of the other" (p. 143). In other words, parents may appear to be poor child managers when they must attempt to control exceptional children. It is not difficult to imagine how the overactive, impulsive behavior of the hyperactive child or the aggression of the conduct-disordered child could quickly elicit very negative responses from the parent. Behavioral observations by various investigators have confirmed the presence of an unusually high rate of coercive interactions within the families of conduct-disordered children (Delfini, Bernal, & Rosen, 1976; Forehand, King, Peed, & Yoder, 1975; Lobitz & Johnson, 1975; Patterson, 1976). As originally described by Patterson (1976), these interactions involve the child's engaging in excessive rates of aversive behaviors followed by parental retaliation with responses that are aversive to the child and are intended to halt the child's behavior. Patterson maintains that whether or not the child halts depends on who escalates his/her aversive behavior more quickly—the parent or the child. If the parent responds quickly with very negative behavior, perhaps some type of harsh discipline, the child may actually halt. This negatively reinforces the parent's use of harsh discipline. If the child's efforts at resisting compliance (yelling, whining, having tantrums) escalate more quickly than the parent's behavior, the parent may give up his/her attempt to make the child comply. This parental acquiescence then has the effect of negatively reinforcing the child's resistance and increases the probability that the child will demonstrate resistant behavior in the future.

Barkley (1981) has speculated that similar types of coercive interactional patterns are observable in the families of hyperactive children. According to his own experience, he says that the mothers of hyperactive children seem most likely to respond to such spirals of aversive parent–child interactions by giving up their attempts to control the child. The parents may even complete the disputed behavioral goal themselves (e.g., cleaning up the child's room or clearing the table), which further reinforces the child's noncompliance. In addition, the mothers of hyperactive children report withdrawing from interactions with their child in an effort to avoid future confrontations. If the child is, on some rare occasion, playing quietly and appropriately, parents report that they do not wish to interrupt this good behavior and may use this time to take care of other household duties. While this parental reaction is quite understandable, it also perpetuates a cycle of behavior in which the child must act out in order to gain the parents' attention.

Lest we end this section on too dismal a note, there is some evidence to suggest that negative parent–child interaction patterns can be interrupted. When hyperactive children increase their levels of compliance, following the onset of treatment with psychostimulant medication, their mothers respond by becoming less commanding and more rewarding of appropriate behavior (Barkley, 1985; Schachar, Taylor, Wieselberg, Thorley, & Rutter, 1987). Even without the use of medication, parents of ADHD and ODD/Conduct Disorder children can be trained to give more effective commands and, therefore, avoid or moderate the creation of cycles of increasingly aversive parent–child interactions (Barkley, 1987; Forehand & McMahon, 1981; Pisterman et al., 1989). And even with adjudicated delinquents, attempts to change family interactional patterns as well as to implement more traditional behavioral contingencies can result in improved family interaction and decreases in antisocial behavior (Alexander & Parsons, 1973; Gordon & Arbuthnot, 1987). The reader is referred to Chapter 2 for more information about interventions to change family processes.

SUMMARY

This chapter has provided a brief overview of the target population for which the intervention described in this book is best suited. While the exact nature of the construct of impulsivity remains a subject of controversy, there is no debate over the fact that children falling into a number of different diagnostic categories display difficulties with impulsive behavior. In summary, it appears that the prevalence rates of hyperactivity and conduct disorder are both approximately 1% to 4% of the population of elementary school children; however, a higher percentage of children display a problematic lack of self-control without displaying all the symptoms of either disorder. The cardinal symptoms of ADHD include attentional difficulties, overactivity, and impulsivity. Other diagnostic groups, such as those with ODD, Conduct Disorder, and/or learning disabilities, may have serious problems with impulsive behavior, but the presence of such difficulties must be carefully determined. Current research suggests that the cognitive deficits of impulsive children are most observable in situations or on tasks that require focused, reflective, self-directed effort. Follow-up studies suggest that there are significant long-term difficulties associated with these childhood problems, including continued impulsivity, poor self-esteem, academic underachievement, and, in some cases, antisocial behavior. The expression of symptoms such as aggression and low self-esteem may also be related to processes within the child's family. Parents and their children may become "locked" in cycles of behavior that perpetuate the child's difficulties, even if parental behavior was not the original cause of the child's problem.

CHAPTER 4

Assessment Issues and Procedures

C areful assessment is a sine qua non for proper intervention. Indeed, the entire assessment process is an information-gathering activity that produces data that better prepare the clinician to make informed decisions. The goal of this chapter is to present an overview of information on a wide range of assessment methods that are consistent with and contribute to information gathering for effective cognitive-behavioral interventions. Clinical settings vary in the breadth and depth of their standard intake evaluations; nevertheless, we encourage the use of several different forms of assessment with virtually every case.

Children who are homogeneous in terms of their impulsivity (or lack of self-control) will nevertheless vary along several other dimensions. For example, one impulsive child may also show severe attentional problems and overactivity and thus qualify for a diagnosis of ADHD, whereas a second impulsive child may not be hyperactive but nonetheless blurts out in class, interrupts peers, and suffers unwanted academic and social consequences. Still another impulsive child may be angry and aggressive, seeking reprisal in situations which, if some thought were applied, would turn out to be minor and unsuitable for retaliation. Although less frequent, still other impulsive children are impulsively compliant. These children seem to follow most rules and appear to do as they are told, but their behavior nevertheless does not benefit from forethought—they act without questioning or thinking about the instructions, the appropriateness of what was asked, or the most efficient manner for follow-through. Even within one of the above clusters, impulsive children will vary along other dimensions, such as level of self-esteem, intellectual ability, and interpersonal skills. A child who is impulsive but has high self-esteem and good peer relations will have treatment needs that differ from those of a child who is equally impulsive but has low self-esteem and poor peer relations. An impulsive child with documented neurological impairments will require very different treatment from an impulsive child who has no neurological signs but has parents who have never been able to set firm and consistent limits. Even if the therapist deemed it appropriate to use a cognitive-behavioral program with most of his/her cases, the varying symptom pictures and histories would demand that the sensitive clinician make some subtle (and probably some not so subtle) variations in the treatment plan for each individual child.

To aid the clinician in gathering useful information and formulating individualized treatment plans, we present a variety of evaluation methods including interview, rating scale, task performance, self-report, behavioral, and sociometric assessment tools. In addition, we briefly discuss naturally occurring archival data that can be useful in developing and evaluating cognitive-behavioral interventions for the impulsive child.

INTERVIEW ASSESSMENT

The intake interview, the most widely used form of clinical assessment, often uncovers pertinent information for any type of intervention. We assume that the clinician already possesses well-developed interview skills, so this section simply includes information that is particularly useful if one anticipates implementing some type of cognitive-behavioral intervention with the child and/or family.

Because the interview process is often used to determine a diagnosis, and because a diagnostic conclusion can also be helpful in making informed treatment decisions, we mention several structured diagnostic interview procedures designed for use with youth or youth and their parents. In general, these structured diagnostic interviews are linked to diagnostic criteria specified in established classification systems (e.g., DSM-III-R; DSM-IV). As a result, the specific questions within the interview schedule may change in accordance with changing diagnostic criteria or the diagnostic system. Users of these or other structured interviews should acquire the most recent edition of the interview and determine that the schedule conforms to prevailing classification schemes. Some of the more commonly used interview schedules include the Diagnostic Interview for Children and Adolescents (DICA) (Herjanic & Reich, 1982), the Diagnostic Interview Schedule for Children (DISC) (Costello, Edelbrock, Kalas, Dulcan, & Klaric, 1984), the Schedule for Affective Disorders and Schizophrenia for School-Aged Children (Kiddie-SADS) (Puig-Antich & Chambers, 1978), and the Schedule for the Assessment of Conduct, Hyperactivity, Anxiety, Mood, and Psychoactive Substances (CHAMPS) (Mannuzza & Klein, 1987).

Parent Interviewing

Along with teachers, parents are, in most cases, the prime source of information regarding the child's behavior and behavioral problems. But parents are typically not mental health professionals and are, therefore, less well versed in the terminology that we use to describe and understand child adjustment. For example, a parent might mention that she has been "depressed." Although this is informative, we do not know if she refers to a diagnostic disorder—depression—or a colloquial term referring to a transient state of being "down in the dumps." Similarly, a parent may use the term *hyperactive*, but without the background information or use of established criteria to warrant or justify the use of the term. Therefore, it is important to help the parent translate terms such as *hyper, out of control*, or *bad* into specific behavioral correlates. For example, hyper might be translated to "he can't sit still at the dinner table" or "he blurts out comments all the time." Bad might be more accurately described as hitting, and more specifically as "she hits her little brother." In traditional behavioral terminology, the antecedents and consequences of these behaviors need to be clarified.

The interview can be used to assess parental expectations for child behavior. For instance, if the parent mentions that the child is hyperactive because he can't sit still at the dinner table, it would be important to also know the expectations that the parent(s) hold with regard to table behavior. Can the child be excused when he is completed the meal? Does "sit still" mean immobile? Or, does it mean staying at the table for a minimum interval? Is a wiggly leg tolerated? Can the children giggle, converse with each other? Parental expectations that table behavior be a rigid adherence to adult-like actions suggest that the expectations, rather than the child, should be a target for change. Equally important is an understanding of the environment of the meal. Is the meal a three-course event that lasts a full hour? Do the parents require that the children sit while they prepare the finishing touches to the meal, sip a drink, or set the table? Is the meal a rush job of five or six different people eating different meals at different times and in various places? Clearly, a parent's statement that "he doesn't sit still at the dinner table" can have multiple meanings and the interview is an ideal setting for acquiring meaningful clarifications.

Obtaining a history of the current problem is also important, and, if the problems are long-standing, the clinician will want to learn why the family is seeking help at *this* particular time (e.g., pressures from the school, marked increases in the child's concern about his/her behavior, additional personal stresses affecting the parents). Also, what have the parents tried in an effort to correct impulsivity? How was it implemented and where was it effective and/or ineffective? Some parents claim to have tried "everything." When such statements are made, the interviewer must encourage the parent to elaborate on each attempted intervention in order to ascertain if the problem is with the intervention or its implementation. The interviewer will also want to be alert to what such a statement may reveal about the parent's belief system and emotional state in relation to the child. Parents who feel that they have tried "everything" without any perceivable impact may be feeling quite hopeless about the prospects for positive change in their child's behavior. This parental sense of hopelessness will need to be addressed early in treatment so that it doesn't limit the potential impact of other treatment efforts that are dependent on having motivated parents. Once the parents regain motivation, the emphasis can be placed on the consistency of rules, the fairness of parental expectations, the affective tone of parent–child interactions, and the follow-through on child effort.

Beyond the discussion of the current problem, we stress the importance of obtaining a developmental history from the parent(s). This information can be crucial in formulating an appropriately comprehensive treatment plan. As part of this developmental history, the mother could be asked about the course of her pregnancy and the birth history of this child, as well as the child's early medical history. The clinician will want to be particularly attentive to factors that suggest possible neurological impairment. The presence of neurologically based problems does *not* contraindicate cognitive-behavioral training, for the child might be in dire need of exactly this type of intervention. Such conditions may, however, require concurrent medical management in order for the child to derive maximal benefit from therapy.

Asking about the child's achievement of early developmental milestones and general temperament as an infant and toddler can yield important information regarding the child's vulnerabilities in certain areas (speech, fine and gross motor coordination, etc.) as well as rich data about the quality of the parent–child relationship. Learning that the parent does not remember when the child spoke his/her first words or cannot recall when toilet training was accomplished would cause the clinician to generate very different hypotheses about the parent–child relationship from those that would be produced by learning that both parents recall each phase of the child's development in detail. Have the parents and child been engaged in power struggles ever since the child could walk? Was the family able to successfully negotiate early separations? Whether or not one values attachment theory, obtaining some sense of how the parent coped with the major events of early childhood can be quite useful, for as Karoly (1981) stated, "The fact remains that adults are frequently the 'creators' of children's self-management dilemmas by virtue of their establishing the task demands and by withdrawing (to varying degrees) their explicit guidance" (p. 105). Discussion of the child's developmental history can provide a convenient framework for discerning how this particular parent tended to establish task demands ("All children should be completely toilet-trained by 18 months" vs. "I figure he'll learn when he's ready") and remove explicit guidance ("My 5-year-old loves to play in the park down the street" vs. "We never let him go into the front yard unless we are with him"). Discussions of developmental history can help to uncover the child's early patterns of interaction. How does the child react to peers—with different peers across the early years? How did the child adjust in school—in different classrooms with different teachers? Consistencies across these various situations can inform the interviewer about the child's (and perhaps the parent's) characteristic interpersonal style.

Finally, the parent interview is crucial for learning what other stresses the family is coping with at this time. Is there chronic marital discord that fosters inconsistent parenting? Fairly consistently, the data support the notion that parent conflict is a major factor in child maladjustment (Emery, 1982; Kurdek & Sinclair, 1988; Shaw & Emery, 1988). Are there special financial or professional pressures on the parents? Is there a seriously ill family member? What is the parent's state of mental health? Research has shown that maternal depression, for example, has a strong impact on how the mother describes the emotional health of her offspring (Brody & Forehand, 1986). Learning of the potential stresses, or the lack thereof, may help the clinician ascertain to what extent the parents are emotionally available to the child or are themselves in need of services.

Child Interviewing

A child is typically brought to see a clinician because some adult (parent, teacher, probation officer, etc.) has deemed the child to be in need of treatment. As we have noted, a child has never called up and said, "Dr. Kendall (or Dr. Braswell), I'm impulsive. Can you help me?" In spite of this adult-oriented state of affairs (or perhaps because of it), interviewing the child can be quite informative. Regardless of whose report is more "truthful," it is interesting to know if the child admits to any difficulties or if he/she sees the problems as they are viewed by parents and/or teachers. Hearing the child's view of the situation will help the clinician begin to discern whether the current difficulties reflect a skills deficit (the child doesn't know *how* to think through a problem or perform the necessary behavior), a mismatch of expectancies (the child can think through the problem and perform the behavior but doesn't recognize what is expected in the problem situation), and/or a motivational issue (the child can think through the problem, perform the behavior, and know what is expected, but there is no reward for doing so or no consequence for failing to do so).

Karoly (1981) suggests that the clinician elicit the child's clarification of an episode of misbehavior by assuming a puzzled or bemused manner and relating some vague details of the event. Typically the child will help fill in the factual details of the setting and the reactions of others, even when he/she is unwilling to describe his/her own role. Even the sharing of small bits of information such as this may tell the clinician about the child's attitude toward the misbehavior (e.g., defiance vs. guilt). Particularly resistant and psychologically unsophisticated children can sometimes be lured into sharing their view of the situation if the clinician recounts a very exaggerated version of the alleged incident: "What's all this about you not doing any homework for a month?" Or, "Did you really beat up your teacher?" "Beat up my teacher, no, I just bop my brother on the head all the time." This technique can backfire, however, and is only recommended for use with some children.

At a more general level, the clinician can assess the child's problem awareness and other existing problem-solving abilities through the use of fictitious stories (Karoly, 1981; Meichenbaum, 1976b, 1977). This method involves presenting the client with a brief story about a child of the same sex who is involved in a problem situation like that of the referred child. With younger children, it may be more comfortable for them to "play out" the story using puppets or dolls. The client can be urged to describe how the story character is feeling and what he/she is thinking in that situation. As recommended by Meichenbaum (1976b, 1977), these narratives can be tape-recorded in order to preserve the sequence of the child's thoughts as well as the content. Examining the content of the child's thoughts, particularly in regard to specific situations, is well within the domain of the cognitive-behaviorist.

Shure and Spivack (1978) have described a process of eliciting the child's thoughts about a particular situation or problem, which they refer to as "dialoguing." Shure and Spivack maintain that via the use of stylistic factors such as a matter-of-fact tone and nonaccusatory questioning, the clinician will be able to carefully guide or direct the child to assess the quality of his/her current methods of problem resolution. As Karoly (1981) points out, this type of procedure blurs the distinction between assessment and intervention; however, dialoguing appears to be a potentially productive mode of interacting with the child in the interview setting.

Our experience dictates that the time spent in a child interview, as well as the time with other assessments, be considered an opportunity to build a relationship with the child. For this reason, as well as the quest for added information, we encourage a playful interview — not a raucous unstructured exchange but a pleasant and fun dialogue. The interviewer can set the desired tone by asking questions with a smile, using references to favorite TV characters, listening to what the child has to say about child-selected topics, and generally communicating that the time with the child is stimulating and that his/her ideas are of merit.

Cross-Informant Inconsistency: Whom Do You Trust?

Early treatment and research in the area of child psychopathology relied largely on parental information. Recently, assessment procedures have called for multiple informants, including children, parents, and teachers

(Institute of Medicine, 1989). As Loeber, Green, and Lahey (1990) noted, however, multiple informants may be challenged because the informants may differ and because there may be differentially appropriate informants for different types of child problems. Loeber et al. (1990) surveyed 128 members of the Society for Research in Child and Adolescent Psychopathology and studied these mental health professionals' perceptions of the utility of children, mothers, and teachers as informants on child psychopathology. The results indicated meaningful variations across types of child problems. For gathering data on the description and frequency of impulsive behavior (hyperactivity, externalizing problems), children's self-report was not considered as important as teacher and parent ratings. In addition to teacher and parent reports, assessments of the presence or absence of thinking skills and the contexts in which these skills are or are not deployed by the child require child-focused assessment as well.

In terms of the data on cross-informant agreement, there has generally been a low to moderate agreement with respect to identifying child symptomatology. Achenbach, McConaughty, and Howell (1987) reported that the relation between informants' reports ranged from mean correlations of .22 to .60. Similar informants (e.g., mothers and fathers) were more highly related (e.g., $r = .60$), while less similar informants provided more disparate reports (e.g., parents/teachers $r = .28$; child/parent $r = .22$). Several factors contribute to such inconsistencies. For instance, the age of the child influences agreement, with older children showing more agreement (Herjanic et al., 1975; Kazdin, French, Unis, & Esvelt-Dawson, 1983). More important for the present discussion, parents reported more externalizing behavior whereas children reported more internalizing symptoms (Edelbrock, Costello, Dulcan, Conover, & Kalas, 1986).

It is our recommendation that parents (and teachers) be used as "outside" observers of the child's patterns of interacting with others, and that there be recognition of and reliance on the child as the reporter of cognitive abilities and emotional states. These later data may come from the child's task performance rather than insightful self-disclosure, but they nevertheless come from the child and not the parent. Multiple sources of information are needed.

BEHAVIOR RATING SCALES

Behavior rating scales provide a global view of the child's behavior as perceived by significant others in the child's environment, usually parents or teachers. Several features of ratings make them particularly valuable to both clinicians and researchers. Rating scales can typically be completed with very little instruction from the mental health professional. They can be completed quickly, and their subsequent scoring and interpretation are rarely time-consuming. These forms also have the advantage of yielding quantitative data (Atkeson & Forehand, 1981; Haynes, 1978). Finally, they do require the rater, whether parent or teacher, to think about the child's behavior in specific terms.

As a result of reading the specific items on the rating scale, the rater may become aware of other problem behaviors that were not included in the initial discussion of the presenting problem (Ciminero & Drabman, 1977). Reading a list of specific problem behaviors may also prompt the rater to reconceptualize the child's problematic actions. For example, we have asked teachers to identify impulsive, non-self-controlled children in their classroom by completing an (SCRS) (Kendall & Wilcox, 1979). One teacher shared that as he began reading the scale items and thinking about a particular child whom he had initially planned to refer, he recognized that while this child did have difficulties, he really wasn't very impulsive. When they are forced to complete a rating scale, raters give more detailed consideration to the child's behavior than they would otherwise.

Many scales are available for use with children presenting the types of difficulties we are discussing. The current review is meant to be illustrative rather than exhaustive. Readers should note the variations in format and focus (general screening measure vs. measures of specific factors) among these scales and select those most appropriate for their client population. In addition to the more standardized rating scales, an example of a more unstructured referral form is presented, as are some experimental uses of cartoons with blank thought bubbles.

Child Behavior Checklist

The Child Behavior Checklist (CBCL) (Achenbach & Edelbrock, 1983) assesses 4- to 16-year-old children's behavioral and emotional problems and their adaptive competencies. The parent completes the scale by indicating which of 118 symptoms or behaviors are descriptive of his/her child now or within the last year. The parent responds to each item using a 3-point scale, with 0 indicating that the item is never true or never occurs, 1 indicating that the item is somewhat or sometimes true of the child, and 2 indicating that the item is very true or frequently occurs. In addition, the parent completes three social competency scales that indicate the child's level of involvement and quality of participation in school, social relations, and nonacademic activities. Each child's scores are then plotted in relation to gender- and age-appropriate (4–5, 6–11, and 12–16 years) norms. The specific number of CBCL subscales produced depends on the age and sex of the child. Factors or subscales that are common to both sexes in age ranges of 6–11 and 12–16 include somatic complaints, withdrawal, hyperactivity, aggressiveness, and delinquency. These authors have also developed a version to be completed by the classroom teacher. Jones, Latkowski, Kircher, and McMahon (1988) reported on norms for 6- to 16-year-old psychiatry inpatients, and Phares, Compas, and Howell (1989) provide data on the relationships between parent (mother and father) and child ratings. Also of interest, Edelbrock and Costello (1988) found meaningful relationships between the hyperactivity score on the CBCL and structured interview diagnoses of ADHD.

While the sensitivity of the CBCL to treatment effects is not yet known, it is a sound method of descriptive classification. Numerous studies have contributed to the positive reliability and validity estimates for this checklist. The CBCL's concern with areas of strength or competency as well as deviant behavior provides a well-rounded picture of the child, as perceived by his/her parents. Knowing about specific strengths could be particularly valuable in treatment planning. For example, if the therapist knows a child excels in a certain subject or recreational activity, he/she can incorporate examples or problems based on the child's area of strength while attempting to introduce a new concept, thus increasing the probability that the child will understand the concept and will remain interested in the therapist's discussion.

The CBCL is recommended because of the age/gender-specific norms that are available, the fact that it looks at psychological difficulties in general, and because it also includes an assessment of the child's social competencies.

Conners Teacher and Parent Questionnaires

The teacher and parent rating scales developed by Conners (1969, 1970, 1973) are perhaps the most frequently used scales for the assessment of hyperactivity in both clinical and research contexts. The parent scale includes 93 items. When factor-analyzed by Goyette, Conners, and Ulrich (1978), the scale yielded the factor grouping of attentional learning problems, psychosomatic problems, impulsive–hyperactive behavior, aggressive conduct problems, and anxious–fearful behavior. Scores on the individual factors can be compared with norms. According to Goyette et al. (1978), individual factor scores do appear to be related to the sex and age of the child. These scores are also influenced by which parent completed the rating, for mothers have been found to report more deviant behavior than have fathers. The teacher questionnaire contains 39 items, but in many hyperactivity studies only the 10 items of the hyperactivity factor are used. This short form·contains items such as "restless or overactive," "disturbs other children," and "fails to finish things he starts—short attention span." Each item is rated on a O to 3 scale and a mean rating is then computed. At an earlier point in time, the standard cutoff for labeling a child hyperactive, when using the 10-item version, was an average score of 1.5. The cutoff is now considered too low, and the abbreviated Conners scale is not a sound method for selecting children with ADHD (see also Ullmann, Sleator, & Sprague, 1985).

Both Conners scales are often used as criteria for subject selection in studies involving hyperactive children, as well as a measure of change in ADHD produced by medications (e.g., Barkley, 1990; Firestone, 1982). While a standardized cutoff point, when employing the full rating scale, may be useful for defining research groups, this method of identifying hyperactive children does tend to yield much higher prevalence rates than other means of subject selection (see "Prevalence" section of Chapter 3). The Conners Parent Questionnaire was found to differentiate between ADHD children and normals (Kuehne, Kehle, & McMahon, 1987), and the Teachers Rating Scale was reported to have acceptable reliabilities (Edelbrock, Greenbaum, & Conover, 1985).

A version of the Conners — called the Iowa Conners — was developed to assess two features of child behavioral problems: inattention/ overactivity and aggression (Loney & Milich, 1982). Normative data on this scale were reported by Pelham, Milich, Murphy, and Murphy (1989). The two scales were reported to correlate .60, but nevertheless evidenced differential validity (Atkins, Pelham, & Licht, 1989). Because each sub-scale consists of only five items, and because there are other scales that are available, the Iowa Conners may be of only limited utility: such as in instances when data are gathered using the larger scale but scores on the two separate factors are of interest.

In one study (Kendall & Brophy, 1981), teacher ratings on the Conners hyperactivity scale were found to be related to other indices of activity (mechanical recordings) but not as meaningfully related to observations of distractibility and attention. The SCRS, mentioned next, was related to both activity and attentional features. For some, there is a trend away from motor activity and toward attentional problems as the central difficulty in ADHD; in such instances the Conners scale may have a limited focus. In addition, the Conners scale typically does not yield information that is particularly helpful in treatment planning, with the exception that hyperactive children who also score high on the anxiety factor may be less responsive to stimulant drug treatment (Barkley, 1977, 1981; Fish, 1971). The frequently used Conners short form covers a very circumscribed range of behaviors and, therefore, is not useful for selecting deficits or identifying treatment-produced changes in other areas of functioning. Although this scale and its variants have been useful in the early studies of hyperactivity, the preferred assessment at the present time is one that includes parent, teacher, and child interviews, standardized parent and teacher behavior rating scales, and direct observational mea-sures (Guevremont, DuPaul, & Barkley, 1990).

Self-Control Rating Scale

The SCRS (Kendall & Wilcox, 1979) was specifically developed to assess the dimension of impulsivity to self-control in elementary school children as rated by their classroom teacher and/or parents (as in Kendall & Braswell, 1982b) (see Figure 4.1). The scale is based on a cognitive-behavioral conceptualization of self-control, wherein self-controlled children are said to possess the cognitive skills necessary to generate and evaluate alternatives *and* the behavioral skills needed to inhibit unwanted behavior and engage in desired action. Of the 33 items, 10 are descriptive of self-control (e.g., "Can the child deliberately calm down when he/she is excited or all wound up?"), 13 are indicative of impulsivity (e.g., "Does the child have to have everything right away?"), and the remaining 10 present both possibilities (e.g., "In answering questions, does the child give one thoughtful answer or blurt out several answers all at once?"). Each of the items is rated on a 7-point scale, and all items are summed to yield a total score. The higher the score the greater the child's impulsivity or lack of self-control. The mean of the SCRS often approximates 100.

When first working on the creation, revision, and selection of final items for the SCRS we sought to include those features of behavior that have been identified in the literature as associated with a lack of self-controlled (impulsive) behavior. For instance, data suggested that impulsive children showed less persistence behavior (Finch, Kendall, Dear-dorff, Anderson, & Sitarz, 1975a), so we prepared an item that would tap observations of behavioral persistence. SCRS item 28 illustrates this: "Does the child jump or switch from activity to activity rather than sticking to one thing at a time?" We also sought teacher input and some of the items reflect their contribution. One item suggested by a teacher was, "If you had but one life to give for your country, it would be this child's." This item does not appear on the scale but its content does provide some information about what some individuals think about impulsive children.

Kendall, Zupan, and Braswell (1981b) found that SCRS scores were meaningfully related to classroom behavior, with higher scores associated with more disruptive behavior in the classroom setting, and Kendall and Wilcox (1979) observed the same relationship in a special testing setting. The SCRS has also been demonstrated as sensitive to the effects of cognitive-behavioral interventions (Kendall & Wilcox, 1980; Kendall & Zupan, 1981; Kendall & Braswell, 1982b) and yields score changes that parallel observed changes in classroom behavior. In one study with in-patient (day-hospital) youth with Conduct Disorder, the SCRS was again found to be sensitive to intervention-produced changes as rated by teachers (Kendall, Reber, McLeer, Epps, & Ronan, 1990).

In addition to distinguishing between non-self-controlled children and normal controls (Kendall et al., 1981b), the mean SCRS score has

Name _____   Grade ____

Rater _____   Date _____

Please rate this child according to the descriptions below by circling the appropriate number. The underlined 4 in the center of each row represents where the average child would fall on this item. Please do not hesitate to use the entire range of possible ratings.

1. When the child promises to do something, can you count on him/her to do it?
   1 2 3 4 5 6 7
   always   never

2. Does the child butt into games or activities even when he/she hasn't been invited?
   1 2 3 4 5 6 7
   never   always

3. Can the child deliberately calm down when he/she is excited or all wound up?
   1 2 3 4 5 6 7
   yes   no

4. Is the quality of the child's work all about the same or does it vary a lot?
   1 2 3 4 5 6 7
   same   varies

5. Does the child work for long-range goals?
   1 2 3 4 5 6 7
   yes   no

6. When the child asks a question, does he/she wait for an answer or jump to something else (e.g., a new question) before waiting for an answer?
   1 2 3 4 5 6 7
   waits   jumps

7. Does the child interrupt inappropriately in conversations with peers or wait his/her turn to speak?
   1 2 3 4 5 6 7
   waits   interrupts

8. Does the child stick to what he/she is doing until he/she is finished with it?
   1 2 3 4 5 6 7
   yes   no

9. Does the child follow the instructions of responsible adults?
   1 2 3 4 5 6 7
   always   never

10. Does the child have to have everything right away?
    1 2 3 4 5 6 7
    no   yes

11. When the child has to wait in line, does he/she do so patiently?
    1 2 3 4 5 6 7
    yes   no

12. Does the child sit still?
    1 2 3 4 5 6 7
    yes   no

13. Can the child follow suggestions of others in group projects, or does he/she insist on imposing his/her own ideas?
    1 2 3 4 5 6 7
    able to follow   imposes

14. Does the child have to be reminded several times to do something before he/she does it?
    1 2 3 4 5 6 7
    never   always

15. When reprimanded, does the child answer back inappropriately?
    1 2 3 4 5 6 7
    never   always

FIGURE 4.1. Self-Control Rating Scale. © 1979, Philip C. Kendall, PhD.

16. Is the child accident prone?

1 2 3 <u>4</u> 5 6 7
no   yes

17. Does the child neglect or forget regular chores or tasks?

1 2 3 <u>4</u> 5 6 7
never   always

18. Are there days when the child seems incapable of settling down to work?

1 2 3 <u>4</u> 5 6 7
never   often

19. Would the child more likely grab a smaller toy today or wait for a larger toy tomorrow, if given the choice?

1 2 3 <u>4</u> 5 6 7
wait   grab

20. Does the child grab for the belongings of others?

1 2 3 <u>4</u> 5 6 7
never   often

21. Does the child bother others when they're trying to do things?

1 2 3 <u>4</u> 5 6 7
no   yes

22. Does the child break basic rules?

1 2 3 <u>4</u> 5 6 7
never   always

23. Does the child watch where he/she is going?

1 2 3 <u>4</u> 5 6 7
always   never

24. In answering questions, does the child give one thoughtful answer or blurt out several answers all at once?

1 2 3 <u>4</u> 5 6 7
one answer   several

25. Is the child easily distracted from his/her work or chores?

1 2 3 <u>4</u> 5 6 7
no   yes

26. Would you describe this child more as careful or careless?

1 2 3 <u>4</u> 5 6 7
careful   careless

27. Does the child play well with peers (follow rules, wait turn, cooperate)?

1 2 3 <u>4</u> 5 6 7
yes   no

28. Does the child jump or switch from activity to activity rather than sticking to one thing at a time?

1 2 3 <u>4</u> 5 6 7
sticks to one   switches

29. If a task is at first too difficult for the child, will he/she get frustrated and quit or first seek help with the problem?

1 2 3 <u>4</u> 5 6 7
seek help   quit.

30. Does the child disrupt games?

1 2 3 <u>4</u> 5 6 7
never   often

31. Does the child think before he/she acts?

1 2 3 <u>4</u> 5 6 7
always   never

32. If the child paid more attention to his/her work, do you think he/she would do much better than at present?

1 2 3 <u>4</u> 5 6 7
no   yes

33. Does the child do too many things at once, or does he/she concentrate on one thing at a time?

1 2 3 <u>4</u> 5 6 7
one thing   too many

been found to be related to other ratings (Reynolds & Stark, 1986) and to vary with the diagnostic category of the child (Robin, Fischel, & Brown, 1984). Hyperactives obtained the highest mean score, followed by conduct-disordered children. Children displaying more internalizing types of problems that did not involve deficits in self-control received the lowest mean ratings (Robin et al., 1984). As noted by Barkley (1990), the SCRS is an instrument that focuses directly on impulsivity—one of the three primary symptoms in ADHD.

The SCRS was originally developed for use by teachers and parents, and both were raters in the Robin et al. (1984) study, with the means for parent raters approximating those for teacher raters. More specifically, Kendall and Braswell (1982b) had both parents and teachers complete the measure and obtained a correlation of .66 between those groups. Similarly, test–retest reliabilities are quite acceptable (.84). Thus, the SCRS can be employed by both teachers and parents. Scores >160 (approximately 1.5 standard deviations above the mean) and <200 are indicative of an impulsive child who is likely to benefit from the intervention program. The extremely high scores often reflect impulsivity as well as a host of concomitant problems that can and often due disrupt treatment progress. Additional research on the development of cutoff scores and the prediction of treatment outcome is needed.

Walker Problem Behavior Identification Checklist

The Walker Problem Behavior Identification Checklist (WPBIC) is a 50-item scale that was originally developed to be completed by the teacher and to assess classroom behaviors that interfere with successful academic performance (Walker, 1970), but it has also been utilized with parents as raters (Christophersen, Barnard, Ford, & Wolf, 1976). This scale presents a two-choice response format that requires the rater to indicate whether a given behavior has been observed within the last 2 months. The problem behavior descriptions are basically straightforward and require the rater to make few inferences. Factor analysis of the WPBIC has yielded five factors: acting out, withdrawal, distractibility, disturbed peer relations, and immaturity (Spivack & Swift, 1973). In computing a child's score, the items are weighted and transformed to standard scores, with a mean of 50 and a standard deviation of 10. Potential disturbance is indicated by a score of 60 or more. The scoring process yields separate totals for each factor, and sex- but not age-related norms for each factor are also provided. Moon and Marlowe (1987) reported the emergence of five factors from their factor analytic study of the WPBIC.

The two-choice response format of this scale may restrict its sensitivity for measuring behavioral change (Kendall, Pellegrini, & Urbain, 1981a), but there is some evidence suggesting that the measure can reflect treatment-produced changes whether it is completed by the teacher (Johnson, Bolstad, & Lobitz, 1976) or the parent (Christophersen et al., 1976). The WPBIC may be useful as an initial screening device that is easily understood by both teachers and parents. In addition, as noted by Atkeson and Forehand (1981), this scale's inclusion of a disturbed peer relations factor, separate from the acting-out and distractibility factors, can provide useful information. For example, considering the current target population of impulsive children it would be helpful to know that a referred child is viewed as distractible by his/her teacher, but that this same rater perceives the child as having few problems in peer relations.

Problem-Oriented Rating Form

In addition to the structured measures described above, it is useful to gather problem descriptions that are more specific to the individual child. Although such information is typically gathered via interviews with the child, parents, and/or teachers, it might be useful to employ a problem-oriented referral form to obtain some information prior to the interview or to use when extensive interviews are not possible. An example of such a form (Urbain, 1982) is presented in Figure 4.2. The information provided by such forms could be very helpful in focusing further assessment efforts and in highlighting specific intervention targets. During the intervention or at its conclusion, the clinician could follow up with a problem-oriented feedback form, such as the one also developed by Urbain (1982) and presented in Figure 4.3.

Assessing Related Constructs: Considering Overactivity, Inattention, and Aggression

As noted early in this book (e.g., Chapter 3), the concepts of overactivity, inattention, and aggression have been implicated in ADHD and share a relationship with impulsivity. The ability to use assessments to separate hyperactivity from aggression has been a question receiving substantial research effort. Using 48 clinic-referred boys and three classroom setting conditions (large group, small group, independent seat), Milich and Fitzgerald (1985) reported that teachers' ratings did discriminate among behavioral patterns. The ratings were obtained on the Conners Teacher Rating Scale, and scores for inattention/overactivity, and aggression, were used in the analyses. The inattention/overactivity ratings were related to behaviors such as failing to attend and failing to comply, whereas the aggression ratings were associated with talking out in class, talking back to the teacher, and being aggressive with peers. As Milich and Fitzgerald (1985) noted, these findings are in contrast to those of Lahey, Green, and Forehand (1980) and may be due to sample differences: Lahey et al. (1980)

Please list, in order of importance, the social behaviors that you perceive as most problematic for this student (PLEASE BE SPECIFIC; i.e., give an example or two if possible).

1. _____

How severe is this problem?

1	2	3	4	5	6	7
Not severe			Moderately severe			Very severe

2. _____

How severe is this problem?

1	2	3	4	5	6	7
Not severe			Moderately severe			Very severe

3. _____

How severe is this problem?

1	2	3	4	5	6	7
Not severe			Moderately severe			Very severe

Please indicate by checking those other specific behaviors you would like to have this child work on. CHECK THOSE THAT ARE MOST IMPORTANT.

____ Taking turns, waiting his/her turn   ____ Listening and paying attention
____ Not hitting   ____ Sharing with others
____ Not pushing   ____ Playing fair (not cheating)
____ Not using offensive language   ____ Not blaming others
____ Not clowning around or showing off   ____ Not teasing or bugging others
____ Not bragging   ____ Telling the truth
____ Staying cool and controlling temper   ____ Not interacting with others; being
____ Sitting still   quiet and withdrawn
____ Communicating feelings more openly   ____ Not bossing and telling others what
____ Compromising more with others   to do
____ Other (specify please) _____

FIGURE 4.2. Problem-oriented rating form.

used nonreferred girls whereas the Milich and Fitzgerald (1985) study used referred boys. It is possible that girls display an overall reduced rate of externalizing problems.

In an elaborate and interesting follow-up study of a large sample of New Zealand children, McGee, Williams, and Silva (1985) conducted canonical correlations of a diversity of ratings and abilities. Cognitive and motor abilities best predicted parent and teacher ratings on inattention.

Below are listed some of the specific problems identified at the beginning of the program. Please rate each according to (1) how severe the problem is at the present time, and (2) level of improvement at this time:

PROBLEM 1 _____

How severe is this problem now? (Please circle one.)

1	2	3	4	5	6	7
Not severe			Moderately severe			Very severe

Has there been any change in this problem since the program began?

1	2	3	4	5	6	7
Got worse	A little worse	No change, about the same	A little better	Improved	Much improved	Very much improved, not a problem anymore

FIGURE 4.3. Sample from a problem-oriented feedback form. *Note.* More than one problem can be listed and the problems can be those on the initial referral form. One can also provide optional space to add any additional problems one would like to have rated.

The Inattention factor identified by McGee et al. (1985) was a behavioral dimension relating to planning, organization, and execution of tasks and activities, and resembled "impulsivity." The Hyperactivity factor consisted of restlessness and overactivity, and the Antisocial Behavior factor also emerged as separate.

Although much of the data seem to converge on the opinion that through careful assessment overactivity, inattention, and aggression can be meaningfully separated, there remains a body of literature that has not found such a distinction to be easy. The question that remains to be addressed is that involving treatment effectiveness: Do the effects of various interventions vary depending on the presence and degree of problems in the areas of inattention, overactivity, and aggression?

Summary

Rating forms, in particular rating scales such as those we have described, can provide some of the most valuable information for making informed decisions. Despite this importance, it must be remembered that such forms are communicating the rater's *perception* of the child, not an actual record of the child's behavior. In some cases, parent ratings may be particularly limited in validity owing to parental misperceptions, parental psychopathology, and/or a lack of exposure to children other than their own. Given this situation, it is highly preferable to obtain ratings from multiple sources whose opportunities to observe the child occur in different settings. Relatedly, rating scales with normative data are preferred over scales without norms. Readers interested in using rating scales that screen for a wide variety of childhood behavior problems are also referred to the literature on the Louisville Behavior Checklist (Miller, Hampe, Barrett, & Noble, 1971), the Personality Inventory for Children (Wirt, Lachar, Klinedinst, & Seat, 1981), and the Revised Behavior Problem Checklist (Hogan, Quay, Vaughn, & Shapiro, 1989; Quay & Peterson, 1983).

TASK PERFORMANCE MEASURES

In this section we describe some of the task performance measures that can be used with impulsive, externalizing, or non-self-controlled children. Before listing these measures, however, we would like to make a few general comments applicable to the administration, use, and interpretation of all the tasks to be described. If administered mechanically with the sole intent of obtaining one score, most task performance measures will yield limited information beyond the one score. But if the examiner is careful to observe *how* the child goes about accomplishing the task demands, information relevant to both diagnosis and treatment can be obtained. Through this type of careful observation, the clinician can attempt to learn about the child's ability to use self-control strategies, capacity for self-direction, and level of metacognitive development, as well as other cognitive abilities.

Metacognition refers to "knowledge concerning one's own cognitive process and products" (Flavell, 1976, p. 232). People demonstrate an awareness of their own cognitive capabilities when they write down a telephone number they must remember, turn off the radio while studying, or repeat to themselves the name of someone they've just met. The examiner can begin to assess the child's metacognitive sophistication through various observations that are readily available in the standard testing situation. As Elkin (1983) noted, virtually any traditional assessment tool can serve the purposes of the cognitive-behaviorist if the examiner is asking him/herself certain questions. When asked to remember a piece of information, does the child employ memory-enhancing strategies or even recognize that he/she needs to use such strategies? If strategies are evident, how sophisticated are they? For example, does the child simply repeat the crucial information or attempt some form of elaboration, such as mental imagery? Does the child seem to recognize the role he/she plays in directing his/her own attention (e.g., talking him/herself through a task vs. requiring direction from an external source)? Also, does the child demonstrate an ability to isolate relevant from irrelevant information in an effort to enhance task performance? How does the child handle frustration with a task? Does he/she talk him/herself through it? Through questions such as these the therapist can gauge, if only subjectively, the child's awareness of his/her own thought processes. Depending on the child's work style, there may be very few clues to the level of sophistication of his/her metacognitive activities. Discerning the degree of awareness the child brings to bear on his/her efforts is often difficult. For example, a child who approaches a problem in a calm and systematic manner may have no awareness that he/she has such an approach. When available, however, this type of information is of special relevance in the implementation of cognitive-behavioral training programs.

As we emphasized in the first edition (see also Loper, 1980), the cognitive aspect of impulse-control training must be calibrated to the child's level of self-awareness. For example, some children may be surprised by the notion that talking to themselves can help them perform better in academic or social situations, while other children already recognize the potential role of self-talk. By keeping these general considerations in mind, the therapist will provide a better match between the intervention and the child. Thus observation of *how* the child does what he/she does on a task performance measure can yield data that are as informative as and perhaps more interesting than a given test score. The following discussion provides illustrations of measures of impersonal problem solving, social cognition, and interpersonal problem solving. If our child clients are going to be apprentices in problem solving, we need to be informed about their current level of general cognitive functioning and their areas of strength as well as those areas in need of special intervention.

Impersonal Problem Solving

A large number of tests have been developed to assess children's cognitive problem-solving abilities. Our present discussion focuses primarily on two measures that have been widely employed and researched with the target sample of interest to us: the Porteus Maze test and the MFF test (e.g., Homatidis & Konstantareas, 1981).

The Porteus Mazes (Porteus, 1955) are a series of paper-and-pencil mazes of graded difficulty that measure aspects of planning ability, foresight, and impulsivity (alternate forms available). The Porteus results in two scores: a quantitative test quotient (TQ) score and a qualitative (Q) score. The TQ score is based on the highest-level maze successfully completed and the number of trials required by the subject to solve each maze. It reflects the child's ability to solve the mazes in the allowed number of trials, independent of the quality of the solution. The Q score is based on the number of qualitative errors, such as lifting the pencil contrary to instructions, cutting across corners in the maze, and bumping into or crossing the sides of maze alleyways.

Porteus originally designed the maze test as an adjunct to early measures of intelligence (Porteus, 1933), as many of the major tests of intelligence have a section that requires maze solution. However, the test has proved particularly sensitive in the identification of non-self-controlled activities seen in delinquency. Interest in the test as a measure of social adjustment, although fluctuating greatly over the years, has reemerged. In fact, Homatidis and Konstantareas (1981) reviewed a number of measures used to identify children diagnosed as hyperactive and found the Porteus Mazes to be one of the better discriminators. As a task, maze performance provides an opportunity for a child to rush, fail to think/look ahead, and display impulsive actions. Careful observation is required.

Riddle and Roberts (1974) reported that the maze test showed acceptable psychometric properties and interrater reliabilities. In their later review, Riddle and Roberts (1977) concluded that the TQ score correlates most highly with tests of visual ability or spatial memory, whereas considerable data indicate that the Q score discriminates delinquents and criminals from normal reference groups. The Q score also discriminated between recidivist and nonrecidivist delinquent groups and is considered the score most sensitive to differences in social adjustment. Keep in mind that recidivism is not easy to predict and that a test that can assist in such prediction is performing quite well. Evaluations of cognitive-behavioral treatments for impulsive, hyperactive, and non-self-controlled children (e.g., Douglas et al., 1976; Kendall & Wilcox, 1980; Palkes et al., 1968) have used the Porteus Mazes to assess changes in the children's planning, judgment, and attentional focusing abilities.

As discussed in Chapter 3, the MFF was developed by Kagan and his colleagues (Kagan, Rosman, Day, Albert, & Phillips, 1964; Kagan, 1966) as a measure of conceptual tempo. A child's cognitive tempo could be determined to be reflective (i.e., slow and accurate) or impulsive (i.e., fast and inaccurate) based on the child's latency to first response and error scores gathered in response to the MFF. The MFF itself is a 12-item match-to-sample task in which the child is shown a single picture of a familiar object and is instructed to select from six variants the one picture that is identical to the stimulus figure. Alternate forms are described in Egeland and Weinberg (1976). When the test is being used for pretreatment, posttreatment, and follow-up assessments, the alternate forms are preferred. These alternate forms consist of eight items each.

Messer (1976), in an earlier review of the reliability and network of correlations associated with the test, concluded that it had strengths and weaknesses. While there are limitations to the instrument (e.g., Ault, Mitchell, & Hartmann, 1976) and some concern about the necessity of including both the latency and error measures in predictions of adjustment and achievement (e.g., Block et al., 1974; Egeland et al., 1980), the MFF has been helpful in assessing impulsivity and evaluating cognitive-behavioral interventions (Bender, 1976; Kendall & Finch, 1976; Meichenbaum & Goodman, 1971). In the Homatidis and Konstantareas (1981) report, the MFF was one of the tests that successfully differentiated the hyperactive from the nonhyperactive subjects. A similar finding was reported in Kuehne et al. (1987). A revised version of this test, the MFF 20 developed by Cairns and Cammock (1978), is reported to have superior psychometric properties. It should also be noted, that while the latency and error scores are sometimes found to both be related to indices of impulsivity and hyperactivity, there are other reports where the relationships hold for one but not the other score (e.g., errors).

The assessor will want to be especially alert to a fast and accurate performance on the MFF. That is, some children who are seen by parents and reported by teachers to be impulsive are not fast and inaccurate but instead are fast and correct. Such a response pattern is not troublesome, as being quick without the cost of inaccuracy is not detrimental. Bright children perform quickly and with a high degree of accuracy, and such success is not associated with detrimental impulsivity. In clinical practice, we have observed that children who are quick yet accurate on tasks such as the MFF tend also to be those children who may not qualify as ADHD and who may not be in need of the impulse control program.

Certain features of both the MFF and Porteus Mazes deserve mention. First, both tests are easily administered in the clinician's office. Second, published data (for MFF norms see Messer, 1976, and Salkind, 1979; for Porteus norms see the test manual and Riddle & Roberts, 1974, 1977) allow the test user to make comparisons of an individual child's score with scores of other children of the same age and sex. Third, both tests provide a sample of the child's behavior in response to standard materials. From the behavior sample, the clinician can make judgments about the child's ability in planning ahead, taking action, and inhibiting unwanted behaviors. Fourth, improvements in these tests may be said to indicate that the child has gained some self-management ability—a more reflective problem approach and a more foresightful test-taking pattern are behavioral samples that reflect an improvement over impulsive and careless performance. Fifth, alternate forms of both tests are available for repeated testing without the unwanted effects of previous exposure to the same stimulus materials.

Recent years have witnessed the development of several computerized methods of assessing ADHD (see Swanson, 1985, for a listing of such programs). Most of the programs include methods of measuring both sustained attention and impulsivity and involve a continuous performance-type task in which the child watches the computer screen for the occurrence of a certain specified stimulus. These measures offer an alternative for sampling attending behavior in the clinical context (Barkley, 1990; Braswell & Bloomquist, 1991), but the data from such instruments are not a replacement for data obtained from other sources and may be less important than actual classroom observations of attending behavior, especially when assessing responsiveness to stimulant medication effects (Rapport et al., 1987).

In addition to the structured tasks, we have sometimes employed more informal questioning to assess impulsivity. The following two examples illustrate the playful style, observing stance, and structured setting that can be useful in getting a handle on the child's impulsiveness. First, questions can be asked to observe impulsive reactions. While playing with a deck of cards, ask the child if he/she would like to see a card trick. The trick, any one of many, requires that the deck be placed on the desk and the child be instructed, "Don't touch the cards." Highly impulsive children are quick to touch the deck—even if the most lilliputian contact is made. Youth with better impulse control can more easily allow their behavior to be governed by such a statement. The assessor can ask the child to "face front and, without turning around, tell me what is behind you." The impulsive child makes a quick turn of the head to try to sneak a peek. Self-controlled children will face forward and try to use memory to recall their ideas of what is behind them. Second, games can be opportunities for informative observation. In checkers, with the rule that if you lift your finger the move counts, impulsive youth are more likely to lift their finger, ask for a do-over, or otherwise try to change an inopportune move. Incidentally, these informal requests can vary and still remain informative, as long as the general principle remains intact: A small rule is stated initially and a violation of this rule could be quick and would seem to benefit the child.

Social Cognition

One aspect of social cognition is the child's ability to recognize the thoughts and feelings of others and to take the perspective of others. Although not receiving much attention in the current research literature, two measures of social cognition that have received research attention in the past merit mention: Chandler's bystander cartoons and Selman's measure of interpersonal awareness. The bystander cartoons (Chandler, 1973) require the child to tell a series of stories based on cartoon sequences presented in picture format. The child is told to pay attention to what the main character is thinking and feeling in each story. After concluding the initial story, the child is asked to retell the story from the point of view of a bystander who arrives later on in the story and is unaware of what happened at the story's beginning. The child receives an "egocentrism" score based on the degree of privileged information ascribed to the bystander (i.e., information available to the child from the previous part of the story, but of which the bystander is unaware). Reliability data are acceptable (e.g., Kurdek, 1977), and there is some evidence indicating significant relationships between the bystander cartoons score and other measures of cognitive perspective taking (Kurdek, 1977) and teachers' ratings of self-control (Kendall et al., 1981b). The relationships among measures of social cognition are not, however, entirely consistent, and some anticipated differences, such as between hyperactive and non hyperactive children, have not been confirmed (Paulauskas & Campbell, 1979). Also, there are powerful influences from level of development on task performance, thus requiring careful consideration of the child's age/cognitive development.

Selman (1980) and his colleagues have developed a series of open-ended interpersonal dilemmas, each of which is geared toward a particular age group and is presented in audiovisual filmstrip format. For example, in one such story, a new girl in town asks Kathy to go to an ice skating show with her the next day. However, Kathy has already made plans to play with her best friend, Becky. To complicate matters further, Becky has already made it clear that she does not like the new girl. An interview follows the presentation of each dilemma. In the case of the sample story just provided, *concepts about friendship* are explored and probed in detail (e.g., how do friendships develop; what makes for good friendship; jealousy). Other dilemmas and interviews serve to examine *concepts about individuals* (e.g., how people get to be the way they are and how they can change), and *conceptions about peer group relations* (e.g., how groups are formed; what makes a good or cohesive group). Each discrete response is scored by comparing it to examples of reasoning at five stages of development. Several indices of reliability have been acceptable (e.g., Selman & Jaquette, 1978; Pellegrini, 1980; Enright, 1977). Initial data support Selman's proposed sequence of developmental stages, and clinic children evidence less mature interpersonal understanding than matched controls (controlling for IQ) (Selman, Jaquette, & Lavin, 1977). While this method of assessing social cognition is interesting, its utility is limited by the extensive training required to master the system and by the questionable status of its relationship to behavior in real-life situations. Nevertheless, the inquisitive assessor may wish to select sample interpersonal situations (tailored to the child's age, nature and context of social dilemmas, and other characteristics) and engage the child in a dialogue about people their age, their friendships, and their interpersonal relationships. The interested reader is referred to Selman, Beardslee, Schultz, Krupa, and Podorefsky (1986) and Yeates and Selman (1989).

Another approach for assessing social cognition involves using cartoons with blank thought bubbles (Kendall & Sessa, in press). Although this approach is still in the developmental phase, it is interesting to speculate about the information that can be gathered. We all have spent time reading the morning cartoons in the newspapers, and we probably have our favorites. Take a select cartoon and white out the thoughts that are in the thought bubbles. Use these cartoons as samples of social situations and ask the child to help fill in the thoughts of the characters. With cartoon sequences that involve social problem settings appropriate for youth, the assessor can begin to see what the child may be lacking in terms of social problem solving.

Interpersonal Problem Solving

There continues to be great interest in measures that assess those skills relevant to solving interpersonal dilemmas along with equal effort to develop programs for training such problem-solving skills (Elias & Branden, 1988; Weissberg, Caplan, & Harwood, 1991). Only a few of the more widely used measures will be presented. Readers interested in seminal theoretical discussions, as well as the role of interpersonal problem solving in adult adjustment, are referred to D'Zurilla (1986), D'Zurilla and Goldfried (1971), Nezu, Nezu, and Perri, (1989), and Spivack and Shure (1974).

We must note, however, that at least some data suggest that the relationship between test responses on some of these measures and behavior in interpersonal dilemmas is modest (e.g., Kendall & Fischler, 1984) and that much of the variance in measures of interpersonal problem solving can be accounted for by assessments of intelligence (Fischler & Kendall, 1988). The interpersonal problem-solving assessment devices to be considered are the Interpersonal Cognitive Problem Solving (ICPS) measures and the Purdue Elementary Problem-Solving Inventory (PEPSI).

Spivack and Shure (1974) and Spivack et al. (1976) have described a series of ICPS skills and developed a series of tests to assess these skills. The ICPS skills include (1) sensitivity to interpersonal problems, (2) causal thinking (i.e., spontaneously linking cause and effect), (3) readiness to consider the consequences of behavior, (4) ability to generate a list of possible solutions, and (5) the ability to generate step-by-step means for reaching specific goals. We note here that the exact steps of this process are not as important as the child's active involvement in some process of thinking through problems and their potential solutions.

Among the measures of Spivack and Shure's skills, means–ends thinking (assessed via the MEPS task) has received the bulk of research attention. One method for the assessment of means–ends problem solving involves presenting the child with a series of stories (typically six) describing hypothetical problems of an interpersonal nature. In each instance, the examiner presents (1) the initial situation and (2) the final outcome, with the child's task being to fill in the middle of the story. Story responses are scored for the total number of means, elaborations of specific means, perception of potential obstacles to carrying out the means, and use of a time sequence.

Means–ends thinking as measured by the MEPS has been found to differentiate between normal controls and (l) a group of institutionalized delinquent adolescents (Platt et al., 1974); and (2) a group of emotionally disturbed 10- to 12-year-olds in a special school (Platt et al., 1974; Shure & Spivack, 1972). In addition to a lower number of elements of means–ends thinking, emotionally disturbed children tended to limit their responses to pragmatic, impulsive, and physically aggressive means (Shure & Spivack, 1972). The means of normals were characterized by greater planning and foresight. Urbain (1979) also reported large differences between impulsive–aggressive second- and third-grade children and a group of nonimpulsive children on a modified version of the MEPS procedure.

The Rochester Social Problem-Solving Group (1978–1979) developed a measure similar to the MEPS, which is referred to as the Open Middle Test (OMT) (see also Weissberg et al., 1991). Each of the four problem stories is accompanied by a series of pictures that the tester displays while explicitly probing for the child's ability to generate multiple solutions. In addition to scoring number of solutions, solution variants, repetitions, irrelevant responses, and chained responses, the child's answer is rated on the effectiveness of the solution and the content categories included. The test authors have reported acceptable interrater reliability for the scoring of responses.

Although seen less often in the literature, tests of alternative thinking and consequential thinking have been developed. The alternative thinking test (see Shure & Spivack, 1978), originally designed for adolescents and adults, has been revised for use with children. The test asks the child to generate as many different solutions as possible to several interpersonal problems (e.g., "how to make new friends"). The awareness-of-consequences test requires the child to consider the pros and cons of an interpersonal action. The test taps more than the simple listing of alternative solutions. The procedure involves describing a story of a child who is in a tempting situation. The child being tested is then asked to "tell everything that is going on in the character's mind, and then tell what happens." Scoring consequences involves the extent to which the child describes what might happen next and the child's weighing the pros and cons before offering a decision (see Spivack et al., 1976).

Use of the MEPS and related measures on interpersonal problem solving, along with other objective measures of behavioral adjustment, allows the clinician to integrate others' ratings of the child's behavior and the clinician's own knowledge of the child's thinking skills in interpersonal contexts. When used clinically, stories with slightly varied content can be added to the standard questions. For example, variations of the MEPS that include peer situations, competitive situations, and academic contexts are worthwhile.

Despite the potential utility of these open-ended measures of ICPS, there are several concerns associated with the ICPS measures and related tests. First, the scoring procedures described in the test manual are not sufficiently detailed and users often create their own additional criteria, resulting in some variability in the scoring procedures employed by different clinicians and researchers. Second, there are a limited number of MEPS stories and an absence of alternative forms, thus making it difficult to conduct both pretreatment and posttreatment testing. In one treatment study, for example, MEPS scores decreased (Kendall & Zupan, 1981) since children, recognizing that they had already answered these questions once, created briefer stories the second time around and, as a result, scored lower. Additional unwanted variability enters into the assessments when different researchers create different stories for the purposes of repeated measurement. Stories that are psychometrically sound for both pre- and posttesting are needed. Third, as previously stated, there is some question regarding the evidence to support the argument that a child's MEPS score actually reflects his/her ability to solve problems in a real-life interpersonal situation (see Butler & Meichenbaum, 1981). The utility of these measures may be enhanced as more is learned about the role of qualitative differences in problem-solving skills and their relationship to adjustment.

Whereas the MEPS is a (somewhat) projective test, the PEPSI illustrates the objective approach to assessing children's problem-solving skills. The PEPSI is a test with 49 cartoon slides that was designed to assess problem solving among disadvantaged elementary school children (Feldhusen & Houtz, 1975; Feldhusen, Houtz, & Ringenbach, 1972). Each cartoon slide portrays the child in a different real-life problem situation. The child listens to an audiotape of directions, problem descriptions, and alternative solutions, and then responds by drawing an "X" in a test booklet over the alternative of the choice. Factor analysis of the PEPSI suggested that it reflects six social problem-solving factors: an evaluative factor and the ability to sense problems, to define problems, to analyze critical details, to see implications, and to make unusual associations (Feldhusen et al., 1972; Speedie, Houtz, Ringenbach, & Feldhusen, 1973). These authors also report acceptable reliability and changes due to a problem-solving intervention. However, the relationship between the PEPSI and indices of behavioral adjustment has yet to be investigated. In addition, since the test uses a multiple-choice format, it precludes the child's generation of alternatives and requires only the selection of a predetermined proper solution. The child's ability to recognize a problem solution is not necessarily the same as the ability to generate a functionally effective solution when no choices are offered. This attribute detracts from the testing being viewed as an indication of problem solving in actual social situations. The test may, nevertheless, be helpful by identifying youth who, as seen in their low scores on the PEPSI, do not recognize the difference between effective and likely-to-be-ineffective problem solutions.

Summary

Performance on various tasks has been used to make inferences about children's abilities: fast and inaccurate performance indicating an absence of forethought and planning; limited generation of alternative problem solutions indicating poor interpersonal problem solving; and interference in storytelling from different perspectives, suggesting deficits in social perspective taking. The large majority of these tasks have been adapted from developmental psychology. While these adaptations benefit from the developmentalist's concern with age-appropriate measurement, many of the tasks were not designed with diagnosis or intervention evaluation as the primary goal. Several of the tasks are essentially projective, and, although they do not seek to uncover intrapsychic conflict, they are based solely on storytelling responses and require the use of complicated scoring procedures. The movement toward more ecologically valid assessments of problem solving (see Rubin & Krasnor, 1984) and social cognition is highly desirable (see section on "Other Analogue Assessments," this chapter). Indeed, assessments that take place in the specific context in question reduce variability due to different situations and, by their nature, are ecologically sound. Thus, while task performance assessments provide an opportunity to witness the child's problem solving in a contrived situation (and perhaps observe an absence of thinking), other measurements taken in real-life contexts are also of value.

SELF-REPORT ASSESSMENT

Earlier in this chapter we discussed the lack of agreement that is often found across different informants of child adjustment. A recommendation that emerges from that literature is that, with reference to self-reports, children with internalizing problems such as anxiety and depression are valuable sources of information on their own emotional state (Kendall, Cantwell, & Kazdin, 1989; Kendall & Ronan, 1990), whereas the value of self-report is limited when one is considering the externalizing disorders such as impulsivity, aggression, and hyperactivity. Few impulsive children engage in self-evaluation, show ability in self-assessment, or provide the necessary reflective thinking for the task of competent completion of self-report measures. Certainly, one would be on extremely weak ground trying to make a determination of ADHD based solely on the child's self-report.

While the child client is rarely used as the sole source of information about him/herself, there are self-report measures that can be quite helpful in specifying the child's areas of strength and weakness and in conveying attitudes or beliefs that may be quite relevant to treatment efforts. We are not using self-report to try to assess the impact of the child's behavior on others, but we can use it to assess the child's expectancies, attributions, and self-concept. These cognitive activities play a role in intervention and an assessment of their level and/or appropriateness before treatment can facilitate individualized intervention.

Expectancies

The view that expectancies influence behavior has been a component of many theories of human learning and behavior (Bandura, 1977, 1986; Rotter, 1966; Tolman, 1932, 1951). The present discussion considers expectations of self-efficacy.

A child's self-efficacy (Bandura, 1977) is the degree to which the child expects that he/she can successfully execute the behaviors that lead to desired outcomes. Changes in self-efficacy have been posited as the common underlying cognitive process that accounts for changes in behavior (Bandura, 1977), and assessments of self-efficacy have been called for in therapy-outcome studies (Kendall, 1982a; Kendall & Korgeski, 1979). Although self-efficacy assessments have appeared in the adult cognitive-behavioral literature, they have yet to receive as much attention in child intervention research. The measurement of self-efficacy involves having subjects state whether they expect to be able to perform certain behaviors (tasks) and how confident they are that they can complete the tasks. Bandura suggests that such efficacy measurement should occur in fairly close proximity to the point when the child will actually be performing the behavior or task.

As an example of such measurement, Schunk (1982) assessed self-efficacy with 7- to 10-year-old children in a study demonstrating that effort attributional feedback for past achievement led to more rapid mastery of new tasks and higher perceptions of self-efficacy. Importantly, children practiced the procedure of rating self-efficacy. A 100-point scale (10-unit intervals) was applied to a jumping task (10—not sure; 40—maybe; 70—pretty sure; 100—very sure). Jumping distances ranged from a few inches to 10 yards. Thus, children were given meaningful experience with the scale and with the notion of estimating confidence. Given that a certain level of cognitive development is necessary for understanding the concept of self-efficacy or confidence, and that children may not be familiar with the standard anchors and descriptions on rating scales, extreme care is required for assessing children's self-efficacy expectations.

Brief assessments of self-efficacy expectations could be included in a traditional testing session. For example, before administering the Porteus Mazes, the tester might ask children whether they expect to be able to solve the mazes and how confident they are that they will complete the task. The child's response to such questions could be quite interesting. One would draw very different conclusions about a child who had no expectation of success yet did succeed, compared to a child who voiced extreme confidence in task performance yet failed, compared to yet another child who requested additional information about the task before voicing any expectations. To return to a point made in the task performance section, this type of questioning is yet another means by which the clinician assesses the child's cognitive and metacognitive sophistication.

Attributions

The concept of attribution is closely related to that of expectancy; however, the two concepts are distinguishable along a temporal dimension (Kendall, 1991b), with expectancies preceding a behavioral event or situation and attributions (i.e., causal attribution) following the event and attempting to specify or account for its cause. To the extent that an individual makes similar attributions across time and situations, he/she is said to manifest an attributional style. Such attributional styles may play an important role in cognitive-behavioral therapy since the explanations that children generate for the behavior and events they anticipate or observe may be a variable that moderates their behavior and the potential effects of treatment.

Assessing expectations of internal versus external locus of control may also yield useful information for the clinician. As discussed by Rotter and Hochreich (1975), persons high in internal control expect events to result from their own actions and attributes, whereas those high in external control expect chance, fate, or powerful others to determine what happens to them.

Several scales have been developed to assess the concept of locus of control specifically in children (e.g., Bialer, 1961). The Intellectual Achievement Responsibility (IAR) Questionnaire was devised by Crandall, Katkovsky, and Crandall (1965) for studying children's locus of control in academic achievement situations, thus limiting the general character of the concept. Another example of a children's locus-of-control measure is the

Nowicki–Strickland Internal–External Scale for Children (Nowicki & Strickland, 1973). This scale consists of 40 yes–no items that are scored in the external direction so that a high score indicates a more external orientation. The Nowicki–Strickland measure seeks to assess locus of control in a generalized fashion rather than assessing expectancies related to only one type of situation. Factor analysis of this scale has yielded distinct factors for emotionally disturbed, delinquent, and normal groups (Kendall, Finch, Little, Chirico, & Ollendick, 1978). This measure has been used to assess therapeutic outcomes, with the results indicating that children manifested more perceptions of internal control following problem-solving training (Allen et al., 1976). A more recent measure is the Multidimensional Measure of Children's Perceptions of Control (MMCPC) (Connell, 1985). The MMCPC is a 24-item scale that measures attributions of causality to internal sources, powerful others, or the unknown.

Children who attribute their behavioral improvement to personal effort may be more likely to show generalization of the improvement than are children who attribute behavioral change to luck, fate, chance, or anything external to themselves. For example, if the child firmly believes that the less impulsive behavior he/she displays is strictly the result of taking medication, it is less likely that this child will even attempt to display the better behavior or control him/herself when not receiving medication. Braswell, Kendall, and Koehler (1982a) obtained results supportive of this hypothesis, with increasing levels of positive change on teacher ratings of classroom behavior associated with attributing positive behavioral change to personal effort. Bugental et al. (1977, 1978) employed an assessment of children's attributions as part of intervention evaluation and reported that those children who had a strong sense of personal control or who were not medicated benefited more from self-control intervention than from a social-reinforcement program.

Children benefit from interventions, and the benefit can be maximized when the child makes sense of the intervention experience and attributes the positive growth to his/her own personal effort. Therapists can be in tune with children's statements about the causes of their behavioral gains and work to shape internal attributions, correct misattributions, and create an atmosphere that fosters the client's capacity for taking credit for personal improvements.

Self-Concept

When an adult refers a child for psychological intervention it is usually reasonable to assume that the goal is to be helpful to the child's adjustment. However, does being sent to a "therapist" have an unwitting negative effect on one's self-definition? Might a child begin to identify with "crazy" people? Stated differently, how does a child referred for evaluation and/or treatment think and feel about him/herself? Do children experience a loss of self-esteem as a result of being "treated"? Self-report indices of self-esteem or self-concept provide information relevant to this question and also provide a means of assessing any treatment-produced changes. Two measures of self-concept will be discussed as illustrations of assessments in this area: the Piers–Harris Children's Self-Concept Scale and the Perceived Competence Scale for Children.

The Piers–Harris Children's Self-Concept Scale (Piers & Harris, 1969) involves a series of true–false or yes–no questions in which the child is asked to indicate what is true for him/her. This questionnaire contains 80 items and was designed to be unidimensional. Factor analysis of this measure has yielded six dimensions; however, the majority of the measure's variance is accounted for by one general self-esteem factor (Bentler & McClain, 1976).

The Self-Perception Profile for Children (Harter, 1985) ia a new revision of the measure originally known as the Perceived Competence Scale for Children (Harter, 1979, 1982). This measure assesses the child's view of his/her own scholastic, social, and athletic competence, as well as behavioral conduct and physical appearance. A global self-esteem scale is also included. One of the strengths of this measure is its innovative response format. In an attempt to avoid the social desirability response set that can affect yes–no types of questionnaires, Harter devised a "structured alternative format." This response format requires the child first to select which of two alternatives is most like him/herself (e.g., "Some kids are always doing things with a lot of kids *but* other kids usually do things by themselves."). After this choice has been made, the child is then asked to qualify his/her response by indicating whether it is really true for him/her or only sort of true. Items are scored on a 4-point scale, with 1 indicating low perceived competence and 4 suggesting high perceived competence. For example, if the child indicated he was most like kids who do things by themselves and then stated this was really true for him, he would receive a score of "1 ." If he chose this same alternative but said it was only sort of true for him he would receive a "2," and so on. This response format is developmentally appropriate — other response formats, such as those that require children to differentiate between "sometimes" and "often," may be too demanding for the youthful respondent.

It is perhaps obvious that these self-report measures, like the several other measures described in this chapter, can help to identify treatment targets or identify factors that may influence treatment effectiveness. A low sense of competence may require competence-enhancing activities, just as a low self-esteem may necessitate extra effort to build more favorable self-descriptions.

Self-reports are also important for the identification of iatrogenic effects. One would certainly want to know if being in an intervention program reduced the children's self-concept. For instance, the therapeutic experiences a child receives may be undermined by a peer context in which participation in the intervention results in a less than favorable nickname for the child. The otherwise positive effects of cognitive-behavioral treatment for impulsivity might be undercut by a child's being goaded by peers, "There's the guy who has to talk to himself!" "Hey hyperboy, can't sit still?" Similarly, if the child learns that some form of treatment is necessary for him/her to be acceptable, he/she could develop an external attributional preference — "I can't do it by myself." Recognition of attributional styles, low levels of self-esteem, or negative self-efficacy expectations are extremely important, particularly when one's goal is ultimately the development of healthy, autonomous individuals. We might mention here, for the sake of completeness, that our data have indicated that children's self-esteem increase as a result of cognitive-behavioral treatment (Kendall & Braswell, 1982b), but we acknowledge that contexts vary in the extent to which it is acceptable for a child to participate in therapeutic activities.

BEHAVIORAL OBSERVATION

Although we encourage the effective incorporation of the assessment of cognitive factors (Kendall & Sessa, in press), we certainly do not intend to discourage or abandon methods of direct behavioral assessment. As a preintervention assessment, behavioral observations can help delineate the problem behavior(s) to be treated and the characteristics of the condition(s) that exacerbate the problem behavior(s). For the evaluation of interventions, behaviors chosen for naturalistic observation should be helpful in the process of specifying what did and what did not change.

Conducting behavioral observations is not without its difficulties. One must first enlist assistants to serve as observers. Training these assistants to reliably assess ongoing behavior in terms of specific codes requires time. Even with adequate training, reliability levels often drop after the initial training period unless periodic checks are conducted. If the child's behavior is filmed for later coding, this adds the concern of potentially expensive equipment. Given these considerations, it is often difficult for therapists to accomplish direct observation of the child's behavior, particularly in naturalistic settings, yet behavioral observations may yield some of the most useful information when working with impulsive-aggressive youth (see McMahon & Forehand, 1988). For example, we discuss behavioral observation systems designed for use in the home and school, but we also present examples of analogue coding systems and the less rigorous, but more practical notion of using the child's significant others as observers. For further information, the reader is referred to Barkley (1990), Karoly (1981), and Mash and Terdal (1988).

Home Observation

One of the most widely known and researched methods of home observation is the Behavioral Coding System (and its variations) developed by Patterson, Ray, Shaw, and Cobb (1969). Within this system, trained observers code ongoing family interaction into 29 possible behavioral categories. These 29 behaviors are classified as either responses or consequences, with the former category inducing behaviors such as command, laugh, touch, and work, and the latter including items such as ignore, approve, and noncompliance.

Typically the family is observed for six to ten 1-hour sessions, with observations occurring during the hour before the evening meal. In order to facilitate these observations, the family is instructed that all members must be present and remain in two adjoining rooms without watching television or making telephone calls. Each member is observed for two randomly selected 5-minute intervals within the hour. During the 5-minute period the behavior of the subject and those interacting with him/her is recorded. The format of this system allows for the examination of the relationship between specific antecedent and consequent behaviors. Readers interested in this type of assessment may also wish to read about a similar system developed by Wahler and his colleagues at the Child Behavior Institute in Tennessee (Wahler, House, & Stambaugh, 1976) and the response-class matrix (Mash, Terdal, & Anderson, 1973; Barkley, Karlsson, Pollard, & Murphy, 1985).

School Observation

A number of observational systems have been developed for use in the classroom. These systems vary in their focus and complexity, but we will describe three examples that are particularly relevant for the current target population. Cobb (1972, 1973) has developed a coding system that concentrates on assessing the child's attentional focusing in structured academic tasks, such as teacher-led discussions and individual work. The 15 categories in this system include behaviors such as attending, talking to teacher (positive and negative), talking to peers (positive and negative), and looking around. One feature recommending this system is Cobb's (1972) report that it can be used reliably after only 4 hours of observer training.

Abikoff and associates (Abikoff & Gittelman, 1985; Abikoff, Gittelman-Klein, & Klein, 1977; Abikoff, Gittelman, & Klein, 1980) presented validational evidence supporting a classroom observational system developed for use in diagnosing hyperactive children. This system includes 10 categories for rating behavior, with the 2 categories of interference and off-task producing the greatest discrimination between hyperactives and normals. Cobb and Hops (1972) developed a coding system specifically for the observation of conduct-disordered children. The 37 behavioral categories of this system fall into eight major headings: approvals and disapprovals, management questions, attention and looking at, talk academic, disruption and inappropriate locale, physical negative and punishment, commands, and miscellaneous. Unlike the two previously mentioned systems, the Cobb and Hops format includes the coding of teacher and peer behaviors that precede and follow the actions of the target child. Thus, as is the case with Patterson's system, one can examine the antecedent and consequent conditions for the behavior of the conduct-disordered child.

Analogue Observation Systems

Given the difficulty of conducting observations in naturalistic settings, some investigators have developed analogue situations designed to mimic selected home and/or school contexts in which inattentive, hyperactive, or aggressive children are likely to have difficulty. According to Atkeson and Forehand (1981), this type of assessment has the advantage of efficiently eliciting the problematic parent–child interactions and providing a standard background against which the clinician can make within- and between-client comparisons. Virtually all of these structured situations are designed to occur in a playroom which can be observed through one-way mirrors.

The Systematic Observation of Academic and Play Settings (SOAPS) was developed by Roberts and colleagues (Roberts, Milich, & Loney, 1985; Roberts, Ray, & Roberts, 1984). Roberts (1990) found that child behavior in the restricted academic setting, as assessed via the SOAPS, reliably discriminated hyperactive, aggressive, and both hyperactive and aggressive boys. Barkley and colleagues also use an analogue system based on a modification of a system originally developed by Milich, Loney, and Landau (1982). As described in Barkley, Fischer, Newby, and Breen (1988), the situation requires the child to complete grade-appropriate math problems while his/her mother reads magazines on the other side of the room. The observation typically lasts 15 minutes and involves rating the extent to which the child is off task, fidgets, vocalizes, talks to mother, plays with objects, is out of his/her seat, and displays negative behavior toward mother. The mother's behavior is also rated in terms of the number of commands made to the child.

Observations by Significant Others

When, owing to concerns with time or expense, the use of trained, nonparticipant observers is impossible, the clinician can enlist the aid of the child's parents and/or teacher as an observer of the problematic behavior. Obviously, given the close relationship between parents or teacher and the child, this type of observation can be subject to bias. It can, however, be extremely useful when attempting to assess low-frequency target behaviors such as setting fires or stealing. Within this area, a number of options are available. For example, several clinicians and researchers working with impulsive youth have suggested that parents and/ or teachers keep a diary of a small number of selected problems for 1 to 2 weeks prior to the intervention. If a more structured assessment is desired, one could prepare a checklist of the key problem behaviors mentioned in the initial interview and ask the parents simply to note the occurrence or nonoccurrence of each problem on a daily basis (Patterson, Reid, Jones, & Conger, 1975). In clinical practice, summer camp counselors, school guidance personnel, and school nurses have collaborated with us in our efforts to gather observations of the child's actual behavior. Almost without exception, these assessments are very specific—only a few behaviors to be monitored—and last for 2 to 4 weeks.

In an effort to gather more information, Wahler et al. (1976) suggest that the parents record the occurrence of, at most, two problem behaviors, but the parents are also asked to note their own behavior preceding and following the child's actions. While the parents' recording of their own behavior may be reactive, it is hoped that this information can be used to analyze the behavioral pattern surrounding the child's inappropriate acts (Karoly, 1981). Because of the reactivity, and because parents want to present in a favorable light in general, it may be necessary for the clinician him/herself to observe the parents' reactions to the child's behavioral problems. These observations can be most informative with regard to tone of voice and other subtle distinctions. For example, one parent reported that she was cuing her son to use his thinking before he made decisions and she described her comments in a manner that was similar to how they were recommended and modeled for her by the therapist. However, when the therapist heard the actual parental comments to the child, the tone was aggressive and threatening, there was no opportunity for the child to comply, and the affective message was condescending, critical, and provocative. Needless to say, the mother reported that she was unaware of her manner of "correcting" her son.

Whether or not one uses nonparticipant observers or the child's significant others, the point is that having some record of the child's actual problem behaviors, as well as the events that precede and follow these behaviors, can be invaluable. We recognize the cost in time and money that is involved in such observation, and we encourage clinicians to develop less troublesome (more creative) methods for witnessing the child in action.

OTHER ANALOGUE ASSESSMENTS

Given the difficulty of conducting observations in naturalistic settings, clinicians and researchers have developed a range of "analogue" assessment methods (Kendall & Norton-Ford, 1982a; Nay, 1986). Analogue techniques can be particularly valuable when one wishes to assess behavior that is important but low frequency, because in the analogue situation one can build in the needed features of the context (e.g., conflict) or provide the opportunities necessary for getting involved in problem solving.

The Structured Real-Life Problem Situation (SRLPS) was developed as a means of assessing the effects of problem-solving training (Allen et al., 1976). This measure involves videotaping an interaction in which the tester and the child approach the testing room, but when they arrive the tester tells the child the room is occupied and cannot be used. The child is then asked to help generate an alternative plan. The child's responses are scored for the number of alternatives produced.

McClure et al. (1978) also designed a real-life assessment situation called the Friendship Club Interaction (FCI). The FCI measure involved children in a "friendship club" contest with the following rules: (1) all six team members must agree on the best answer to the contest questions; (2) all six members must help answer the questions; and (3) all six members have to be club officers. A number of actual problems were present in the setting, such as five chairs for six subjects, five officer possibilities for six subjects, and the problem of distributing officer titles. The problem-solving interaction was videotaped and coded for problem-solving responses. With both the FCI (McClure et al., 1978) and SRLPS (Allen et al., 1976) measures, subjects who had received problem-solving training obtained higher scores than control subjects.

A variety of research studies have adopted a method of assessment that includes discussion of conflict or disagreement. For example, some efforts to examine interpersonal cognitive problem solving in an analogue context have involved the child and parents, with each being asked separately to think of ways to spend a sum of money and then being brought together to discuss methods that could be used to resolve any disagreements. Others, studying the behavioral interaction patterns of adolescents and their parents, have created a similar context and asked the participants to discuss how to resolve previously identified matters of conflict between the youth and his/her parents.

These creative efforts at skills assessment are laudable, although, for the practicing clinician, recommendations for videotaping such interactions and later rating them on various dimensions could be as time-consuming and impractical as actually conducting naturalistic observations. It would be possible, however, for most clinicians to include opportunities for the child to attempt solving at least minor real-life problems in a standard evaluation. Finding the testing room (bathroom, drinking fountain, etc.), having too few chairs in the testing room, opening a locked cabinet or desk drawer, borrowing necessary equipment from others — these are all situations in which the clinician can informally assess the child's problem-solving style, manner of addressing conflict, and style of coping. In addition, the clinician could ask families to audiotape attempts to discuss family problems at home and then bring the tapes to the clinician for review.

The clinician may also want to role-play problem situations that are reported to be trouble spots for the child. Role plays can serve the purposes of both assessment and treatment. Keep in mind, however, that research by Beck, Forehand, Neeper, and Baskin (1982) suggests that role-play situations may elicit more social behaviors than are observed in similar but more naturalistic interactions. They hypothesize that interacting with an adult therapist who provides social prompts may be easier for some children than interacting with peers, so that role-play situations may present a more positive view of the child's social abilities. With this caution in mind, therapist–child role plays may still prove valuable if one is concerned with how the child can behave under optimal conditions. For example, if the child cannot generate and display some appropriate responses for, say, conflict resolution or initiating play even when interacting with the therapist, this may give some indication of the severity of the deficit.

SOCIOMETRICS

A child's ability to interact with his/her peers yields important information, because children are remarkable judges of their peers' adjustment (e.g., Cowen, Pederson, Babigian, Izzo, & Trost, 1973). Sociometric assessment provides some indication of the child's social standing and level of peer acceptance. Unfortunately, few clinicians are able to avail themselves of this information because of the time and out-of-office activity required to obtain it. We will, however, briefly discuss the more common methods of obtaining sociometric ratings, in hopes that the interested reader may someday be able to pursue this area.

The vast majority of sociometric assessment methods can be classified into one of three major types. The peer-nominations approach is perhaps the most direct and simple method of assessing sociometric status. This type of assessment requires children to nominate their peers for inclusion in some group (e.g., Whom would you like to play with? Whom would you like to work with?). An even more direct version of this approach simply asks children to choose whom they like most and least (Busk, Ford, & Schulman, 1973; Roff, Sells, & Golden, 1972).

Rating scales have also been applied to sociometric assessment. Typically, with this approach children are provided a list of their classmates' names and asked to rate each on some dimension of acceptability (e.g., How much do you like to play with this person at recess?). Examples of this type include the Ohio Social Acceptance Scale (Lorber, 1970).

The third approach is referred to as "descriptive matching," or type-casting, for the children are asked to match up peers with various behavioral or personality descriptors. For example, with Bower's (1969) Class Play, children are asked to assume the role of director and cast their peers for any of 20 roles in an imaginary class play. Importantly, Class Play was developed specifically for the early identification of maladjustment in schoolchildren.

The exact nature of what is being measured by sociometrics (the characteristics of others or one's own feelings about them) and the degree of confidence one places in peer assessments remain a source of discussion (Brief, 1980; Kane & Lawler, 1978). Nevertheless, sociometric status tends to be a stable variable, in the absence of intervention, and sociometric assessments have proved sensitive to emotional maladjustment in regular schools. Bower (1969) reported that children with clinical problems, unbeknownst to teachers and classmates, tended to be chosen for negative, hostile, or inadequate roles, or not chosen at all for Class Play.

ARCHIVAL DATA

Certain real-world measures that accrue in archives can offer information important to a full understanding of the child's problems, as well as provide convincing evidence for treatment effectiveness. The most obvious examples include information such as grades, past achievement test scores, and records of "visits to the principal," which could be obtained from the child's school record if a teacher interview is impossible and the child's parents give their permission to open the school file.

In terms of treatment evaluation, Chandler (1973) and Alexander and Parsons (1973) documented the impact of their interventions with delinquents using recidivism data. Moreover, Klein et al. (1977) reported reduced recidivism among treated subjects and their siblings. Similar measures can be profitable in the context of a school intervention. For example, Sarason and Sarason (1981) assessed the effectiveness of a social–cognitive intervention with adolescents at risk for dropping out and delinquency by counting the rates of tardiness, absence, and referral for misbehavior in the year following the intervention. A cognitive-behavioral intervention with aggressive children might be evaluated in terms of the number of detentions or formal reprimands received during a subsequent grading period or the next year. A more academically oriented intervention could examine the child's actual grades in the treatment-relevant courses. As obvious as these types of measures seem, they have yet to be fully integrated into evaluations for cognitive-behavioral treatment.

GENERAL CONCERNS

In any intervention, one must be concerned with the *levels* of assessment. Two levels of assessment have been described by Kendall et al. (1981a): the *specifying level* and the *general impact level.* At the specifying level, the evaluator is interested in determining exactly what behaviors or processes are problematic for the child. Measurement at this level helps the professional focus on what may need to be changed and provides the data necessary to determine precisely what did or did not change as a result of any intervention efforts. What exact skills were found to be lacking and were acquired, and what specific detrimental behaviors were observed initially and were later found to be modified? The key to the specifying level is that specific skills and specific behaviors be assessed.

In contrast, general-impact-level assessments are sought not to specify what exactly needs to be changed, or what did or did not change, but to determine the general impact of the child's behavior on those around him/her. How is the child perceived by peers, teachers, or parents? Is the child perceived differently as a result of treatment? Appropriate assessments at the specifying level include behavioral observations, task performance measures, and indices of specific cognitive processes. Teacher and parent ratings, sociometric assessments, and archival data are examples of general-impact-level assessments. Use of *both* specifying and impact-level assessments, and measuring both cognitive and behavioral change, would aid the clinician in understanding the child's specific deficits and assets and in understanding how the child is perceived in his/her social world.

At a more practical level, we realize that not all therapists have the luxury of extended evaluations that include parent, teacher, and peer ratings as well as all relevant psychometric information. We believe, however, that the concepts emphasized in our discussion of these various measures could be incorporated into the format of one's standard procedures. Gathering information about the child's impersonal and interpersonal problem solving is valuable, and there are myriad ways in which this information could be obtained.

The focus of this chapter has been on the assessment of the cognitive and behavioral functioning in the child and our goal has been to better understand the nature of the child's difficulties. However, one could easily turn the assessment task over to an examination of the family (parents). What are the contingencies in the family environment? What family interaction patterns are consistent and detrimental to the child's developing into an independent and thoughtful adult? Is there any evidence of cognitive, emotional, or behavioral psychopathology in either or both of the parents? Are there other contextual issues that serve to maintain the child's maladjustment?

Currently, there is not a diagnostic category that identifies the family (and not the child) as maladjusted or disordered (Kendall & Morris, 1991), and there are few easily administered and psychometrically sound measures of family functioning that have direct influence on impulsivity in the child. Nevertheless, the assessment of family factors cannot be ignored. Inaccurate attributions on the part of a parent (my child gets upset because he is ADHD, instead of, he gets upset because that is normal for youth in that situation), as well as unrealistic expectations (he should be able to sit still for the family meal—even if it lasts 50 minutes and he is finished with his meal) can contribute to both the development and the maintenance of perceived child maladjustment. Gathering some information about the parents, about the family interaction pattern, and about the social context provides the required backdrop against which to examine the data from assessments of the child.

Once the information is in hand (or, more accurately, in mind), the clinician can then engage in his/her own information processing in order to decide whether this child's difficulties are, in fact, appropriate for remediation with the cognitive-behavioral methods described in this book. If the answer is yes, the clinician is ready to use the available data on the child (and on the relevant intervention techniques) to formulate a specific treatment plan. We strongly recommend the preparation of a treatment plan or outline for each child. We view this as an aid to the therapist's own problem solving as he/she directs or guides the activity of each session. The reader is referred to Braswell and Bloomquist (1991) for added discussion of the matching of specific cognitive and behavioral targets with specific intervention techniques in the formulation of a treatment plan. Assessments are highly valued because they provide data for gaining a better understanding of the person, making informed decisions, and facilitating the individualized treatment plan.

CHAPTER 5

Treatment:
The Basic Ingredients

The separate strategies that combine to form cognitive-behavioral therapy for impulsive children are described and illustrated in this chapter. Our intent is to provide both a general description of each of the strategies and some sample transcript materials. We recommend the following sections, even to the reader who is already employing some of the suggested strategies, because our discussions of strategies and transcripts of case materials illustrate not only correct and successful application, but also areas in which difficulties arise and in which some recommended remedies may be undertaken.

The main strategies used within cognitive-behavioral therapy for impulsive children include (1) a problem-solving approach, (2) self-instructional training, (3) behavioral contingencies, (4) modeling, (5) affective education, and (6) role-play exercises. Recommendations for tasks to be used in training are also provided. The treatment strategies are essentially an interwoven program that can be implemented using the *Stop and Think Workbook* (Kendall, 1992a), but, for the sake of ease of description, we will present each strategy in a separate section and describe the *Stop and Think Workbook* at the end. Readers interested in the detailed and systematic description of the program are referred to the treatment manual (Kendall, 1992b) as well as to the videotape (Kendall & Braswell, 1982c) available from the first author.

PROBLEM-SOLVING APPROACH

Fundamental to the strategies we will be discussing is an underlying problem-solving theme. Our focus is on interpersonal problems, although the skills that are useful for interpersonal problem solving can be acquired through practice with both impersonal and interpersonal problems. When we use the term *problem solving* and ask about problem-solving skills we are asking questions like the following: What are the cues that people use to recognize when there is an interpersonal problem? What are the options available for working toward solutions to interpersonal problems? What are the likely consequences associated with various alternative solutions? When we begin to consider the features of interpersonal problem solving, we soon realize that the more accurate descriptive label for our approach is social–cognitive problem solving. It is an approach that strives to remedy deficiencies in cognitive functioning by teaching cognitive strategies for interpersonal problem solving.

Why Problem Solving?

Our answer is simple: because problem-solving skills are required for successful psychological adjustment. Jahoda's (1953, 1958) early writings discussed the relationship between interpersonal problem solving and social and emotional adjustment. Accordingly, psychological health is related to a problem-solving sequence consisting of the ability to recognize and admit a problem, to reflect on problem solutions, to make a decision, and to take action.

More recent advances in the theory and application of problem-solving approaches to treatment were made as a result of D'Zurilla and Goldfried's (1971) identification of problem solving as a component of behavior therapy. These authors defined a problem as a situation to which a person must respond in order to function effectively but for which no effective response is readily available. D'Zurilla and Nezu (1982), Spivack and Shure (1974), Weissberg, Caplan, and Harwood (1991), Elias and Branden (1988), and Rubin and Krasnor (1984) have further elaborated on the process of social problem solving, the relationship of social problem solving to psychological dysfunction, and the current status of the assessment and training of social problem-solving skills. Given that maladjustment can be viewed as ineffective responding, and that maladjustment typically involves ineffective problem solutions, the central role of problem-solving skills in adjustment is readily recognized. Like it or not, we all encounter problems that require solutions. Impulsive children are no exception; they do differ, however, in that they routinely lack the skills in problem solving needed to produce adaptive solutions.

Why Cognition?

The full range of possible solutions to problems typically does not materialize from thin air, nor does the single best solution necessarily pop into one's head first. Rather, successful problem solving results from an involvement in the operation of cognitive strategies that allows the person to consider possible courses of action, reflect on potential outcomes, and make decisions about options. Some individuals seem to reach the best solution in an errorless and energyless fashion, but don't be fooled. Optimal solutions may "pop" out on some occasions, but the first idea is not always the best. Much thought often precedes a decision, and a thought-out decision is more often one that can be lived with by the parties involved.

An important component of problem solving, whether interpersonal or impersonal, is the cognitive processing of relevant information. Information-processing theories reflect the assumption that the theory can be translated into an executable program and that there is correspondence between the temporally ordered states of the human process described by the theory. In addition, the output that is reached as a result of the input that is provided depends on the skill base and knowledge state of the information-processing system. Information-processing analyses are valuable guides to our understanding of what is involved in interpersonal problem solving.

Several writers have applied cognitive information-processing ideas to clinical psychology (see Ingram, 1986). For example, Beck's theory of the role of cognition in depression (1976) illustrates one link between information-processing science and clinical psychology. More recently, the complex nature of cognitive functioning has been elaborated and applied to several areas of psychological distress. For instance, it has been suggested (Ingram & Kendall, 1986; Kendall & Ingram, 1989) that cognitive content (events), processes, products, and structures can be distinguished. The central notion here is that cognition is not a singular or unitary concept.

Cognitive structures can be viewed as memory, including the manner with which information is stored in memory. Through experience, individuals develop a structure which in turn influences how future events are experienced. Cognitive content refers to the information that is actually represented in memory: the content of the structure. Content also refers to the surface-level statements that one makes when identifying the thoughts that are on one's mind: the content of the thinking at that moment. Cognitive processes are the procedures used to operate the cognitive system. Cognitive processes refer to the manner in which we perceive and interpret experiences. Cognitive products are the cognitions that result from the interaction of incoming information, cognitive content, cognitive structures, and cognitive processes. Statements reflecting causal attributions are examples of cognitive products, for as we struggle to disambiguate the causes of behavior we reach attributional conclusions.

Cognitive structures can be called templates—for they are an accumulation of experiences that serve to filter or screen new experiences. An angry and aggressive child has a history of being yelled at for his behavior and brings this history to new experiences. When the pot is found broken, he may be first to say he didn't do it. From his experience, he feels the need to defend himself. An impulsive child is likely to have a limited history of using cognitive problem solving to his/her advantage and will, accordingly, not yet know the benefits of employing a cognitive structure (template) for seeing situations as simple problems to be solved. Speaking in terms of treatment, cognitive-behavioral therapy for impulsive children seeks to provide experiences that allow for rehearsal of cognitive content that includes processing that is useful for solving problems, and strives to build a template that includes "coping." Impulsive children can benefit from learning a series of self-directed statements that can inhibit fast action, guide one toward problem resolution, and, in the end, include a pat on the back for successful coping. The goal is not a template that is errorless but one that has a means for coping with the inevitable challenges and errors that are before us.

Cognition is especially critical when children are the target sample because of the large-scale developmental changes and influences that take place. For instance, Piaget (1926) offers meaningful contributions about cognitive functioning that have implications for matters of intervention. Piaget's approach is very much concerned with how an individual's cognitive structures both shape and are shaped by the person's interactions with the environment. Accommodation and assimilation are concepts that illustrate this aspect of Piaget's theory. With the presence of certain underlying cognitive structures, the person's interactions with the environment affect the cognitive structures and the person's behavior. The structures are not stagnant.

Developmental influences also affect cognitive processing. Gal'perin (1969) described a developmental series of events leading to the eventual automaticity of cognitive processing. The importance of this theoretical model is that it outlines the steps that a therapist would want to follow to successfully teach the desired mental activity and have it become automatic. The first step involves familiarization with the task. Next, the person performs the task on the basis of its material representation. This step is followed by performance acts explicitly related to overt speech, and subsequently the external speech is self-directed. The culmination of the process is reached when the act is completed using internal speech alone.

It seems reasonable to assert that since there exists an indefinite number of potential problem situations and an infinite list of discrete solutions, interventions are best focused not on teaching specific responses but on *training the cognitive processes* involved in problem solving. The ability to achieve successful problem solutions across various situations is the desired therapeutic outcome.

Why Social?

The type of problem solving that is of present concern has to do with effective coping in social situations — social or interpersonal problem solving. A child's ability to excel in *impersonal* problem solving is not necessarily related to arriving at solutions to *interpersonal* or social problems. There is essentially no strong evidence to support an assumption that impersonal and interpersonal problem-solving skills tap the same cognitive structures or processes, or that individuals who readily solve impersonal problems necessarily are similarly competent with social situations. One reason for the social focus, then, is that the problems seeking solutions have to do with peers, siblings, teachers, and family members. Such problems are inherently social.

Many of us can recognize "good" social problem solvers, and some of us sometimes suffer from the errors of those lacking such skills. Nevertheless, we have not yet reached a complete understanding of the process of social problem solving. Most studies assess the repertoire of abilities necessary for good problem solving and several studies go on to compare distressed and nondistressed subjects' performance. Typically, the procedures used require subjects to describe potential problem solutions. What is needed are studies of the plans that are followed, the strategies that are employed, and, especially important, the thinking processes that guide accepting or rejecting potential problem solutions.

A second reason for the emphasis on "social" is based on the apparent critical role of the social context for successful development. Wide agreement exists that satisfactory relations with peers is a crucial component of children's successful adjustment to life. Poor peer relations early in life have been reported to have serious effects on later adjustment. For instance, Robins (1966), Roff (1961), and Cowen et al. (1973) all provide evidence that suggests that negative social standing among peers is a critical precursor of adult psychopathology. Research with rhesus monkeys (Harlow & Mears, 1979) has demonstrated a strong relationship between negative states and a lack of social experience, leading the authors to conclude that isolation without social interaction has serious, if not disastrous, effects. Interestingly, these authors also report that social contexts (peers) are powerful factors in rehabilitation (see Hartup, 1983).

Regarding the intervention strategies per se, therapists want to keep the training context as close as possible to real life. Since many interventions are designed to stimulate the cognitive processes associated with real problem solutions, it seems reasonable to propose that they be taught in the interpersonal situations in which problems arise. Thus, while the therapist–child relationship may be an adequate context for initially introducing new skills, training should move beyond this context to include practice in problem solving with parents, siblings, teachers, and peers.

An additional consideration comes to the foreground when we return again to the larger question: Why social–cognitive problem solving? We are, as are many current child therapists, influenced by behavioral psychology. The result is that interventions are intended to teach abilities and/or remedy skill deficits, and it is through *performance-based* procedures that such goals are reached. We refer here also to the fact that interventions are enhanced when the proper contingencies are arranged to motivate and reinforce learning. However, behavioral strategies place too great an emphasis on training discrete observable behaviors and all too often ignore the cognitive components of effective adjustment. Social–cognitive problem solving becomes the major focus, for it is concerned with teaching component problem-solving abilities and the cognitive processes associated with behavioral adjustment, all within the realm of the child's social environment. It is a purposeful amalgam, maintaining some of the demonstrated virtues of behavioral therapy but expanding them to envelop a larger domain of relevant cognitive and social functioning.

SELF-INSTRUCTIONAL TRAINING

We propose that an effective means to the solution to a problem is via the careful examination and execution of the problem-solving process. Self-instructions are self-directed statements that provide a thinking strategy for children with deficits in this area and serve as a guide for the child to follow through the process of problem solving. Self-instructions reflect the desire of the therapist to break down the process into discrete steps, and, accordingly, each self-instruction represents one step of solving a problem.

In various research reports, discussions, and chapters, self-instructions have been illustrated as in Table 5.1. As shown, the content of the self-instruction includes five types of statements. These self-directed statements proceed from (1) the generation of a problem definition, to (2) stating the problem approach, (3) focusing attention, and (4) self-rewarding for correct responses. Following incorrect solutions, (5) coping statements are used to help teach the child that all is not lost, that he/she

TABLE 5.1. Content of Self-Instructional Procedures

Problem definition:	"Let's see, what am I supposed to do?"
Problem approach:	"I have to look at all the possibilities."
Focusing of attention:	"I better concentrate and focus in, and think only of what I'm doing right now."
Coosing an answer:	"I think it's this one . . ."
Self-reinforcement: or	"Hey, not bad. I really did a good job."
Coping statement:	"Oh, I made a mistake. Next time I'll try to go slower and concentrate more and maybe I'll get the right answer."

Note. After Meichenbaum and Goodman (1971); Kendall (1977); Kendall and Finch (1979b).

can try again, and, above all, that committing an error does not necessitate
a disturbing outburst. Coping self-talk is intended to help the child
develop greater tolerance for frustration—when things don't go well, it's
OK to stop and try again. We describe self-instructional procedures in as
clear a manner as possible, but we also acknowledge that employing
self-instructions is not as simple as it may seem at first reading. We direct
readers to pay special attention to the ideas that govern treatment implementation that are described in Chapter 6.

The problem-solving self-instructions are designed to help the child
(1) recognize that there is a problem and identify its features, (2) initiate a
strategy that will help him/her move toward a problem solution, (3)
consider the options, and (4) take action on the chosen plan. Importantly,
the self-rewarding self-instruction is included to strengthen the child's
"thinking" habit. When errors are made, the coping statements are designed to avoid overly negative self-talk. We do not want children to try,
to make a mistake, and to tell themselves, "That was really stupid; I'm
dumb," get frustrated, and give up. What we do want is an effort, and, if
the effort proves incorrect, a comparatively neutral self-stated reaction
such as, "Oops, I made a mistake. I'll have to think it over again."

One of the most important aspects of the self-instructional procedure
is the meaningfulness of the actual sentences for the individual child. That
is, saying the self-instructions the way we therapists would *is not* as crucial
as having the child say them in his/her own words. The therapist and child
collaborate to create (have the child discover) specific self-directive statements. Individualizing the self-directed statements far surpasses "saying
what we say" as the goal of the therapist. Indeed, in the first "Stop and
Think" session the therapist and the child collaborate to create "the steps"
(the self-directions) and write them down on the back of the stop sign that
later serves as the bookmark for the workbook. The following transcript
illustrates not only the self-instructional training procedure as outlined
thus far, but also the individualizing of the problem-solving self-
statements.

Therapist: Now, when we do these tasks I am going to show you how we
think out loud while doing them, OK?

Child: All right.

T: I'm going to do the first one, and you can look over and watch as I do
it. Now there are several steps to follow. Notice that when I say the
first step, then I do the first step. Now the first one is, "What am I
supposed to do?" Well, I'm supposed to, according to this task, find
out which one comes next. Do you see what I mean?

C: Yeah.

T: OK, my next step is look at all of the possibilities. Boy, there are a whole lot of things on this page. The next step is to focus in; I guess that means I don't need to look at these other problems on the rest of this page, I just need to look at this one. Now, the letters are Q, S, and U. . . . And, the task was to find which one comes next. So, it seems to be letters, skipping to every other one. The next step is picking the answer, OK?

C: All right.

T: There is a lot to remember, isn't there?

C: Yeah.

T: OK now, Q, R, S, T, U, V, W. So, the one that comes next is W. Then, when you get the problem right—and we agree that W is the right answer—when you get it right you say to yourself, "I did a good job." If you get it wrong, then it is sometimes a good idea to say to yourself, "Next time I've got to go more slowly and try to think more carefully." So, that's how I used the steps. Now might you do it? Want to try?

C: All right.

T: Seems like a lot though, doesn't it?

C: Yup. Do I have to learn them all right away?

T: No, we can take our time. We'll work on them together and go slowly. You don't have to learn them all exactly the way I said them, you can use the steps you want. OK, why don't you try and do the next one, and as you do it let's start to write your own ideas down for things to say for each step. I'll help.

C: All right.

T: What is the first step? Here, you can read my list.

C: "What am I supposed to do?"

T: Great. OK, now how would you say that in your own words? How would you say to yourself, "What am I supposed to do?"

C: "What is the problem?"

T: Good. OK, that's a great way to say it. "What is the problem?" It lets you know that there is a problem to work on. Why don't you write that here on the back of the stop sign. You can go ahead and do that. We'll put the steps that you design on this stop sign and you can use it to remind yourself later. (Pause) Good job. "What is the problem?" OK, now that we've said it, let's do it . . . what is the problem for that one?

C: I've got to find the answer.

T: OK, and how is this problem defined, what is it that is the answer?

C: Which one comes next?

T: Exactly. So that's the problem: Which one comes next. The second step was, "Look at all the possibilities." That's the way I said. Do you know what possibilities means?

C: Choices?

T: Yeah. Good. So, how would you say this step to yourself. How would you say, "Look at all the possibilities"?

C: "Look at all the choices."

T: Excellent. OK, you can write that step here. You wrote "choices." OK, that will be a good way to remember to look at all the choices. Want to draw some big eyes over here—to suggest looking at the choices?

　　Now, the next step is to focus in. You don't need to look at the ones at the bottom of the page, so you might block those out. OK. Now, what would be a way that you would say to yourself to focus in?

C: To look at just these ones.

T: OK, good. What would be a way you'd say that to yourself? What would be a way you might say that? Just look at these?

C: "Focus in."

T: OK, sure. Then why don't you go ahead and write that right here. To focus in is sort of like thinking really hard. You've got to focus in and think hard. Good. All right then, the next step that I used was "pick an answer."

　　So far we went through these real quick. Let's go back over them again so you can do them when you say them. No hurry, let's take our time.

　　What is the problem? Now, what is the problem in this case?

C: Which number comes next?

T: OK. The second step was "choices," and then "focus in." Why don't you say and then do each of those. (then, said as if to self) "Focus in and look at the choices."

　　Now, think about each choice, and which one might be the right answer.

　　(Pause) The next thing you are supposed to remember is to pick an answer. Which one do you pick?

C: Ten. Cause it goes 1, 4, 7, and then add three and you get 10.

T: OK, let me check. That is right. When you say "pick an answer," how do you say that to yourself?

C: "Pick the right one." Or maybe pick the choice.

T: Pick the choice, OK. This is good. Pick the right choice, or pick the choice. Now, you got that one right, and when you get it correct what would you say to yourself?

C: "I did a good job."

T: OK, that's what I said, too. How do you say that to yourself when you do something really well? How do you say that to yourself?

C: "I did a good job."

T: So, that's how you'd say it too.

C: Mm.

T: OK, so we'll just keep that the same. Let's write it on your stop sign. Go ahead and put it in your own words.

  Now we have all the steps that you can use when we work on problems. This may seem like a lot to learn, but we are going to have plenty of time to practice and, you've got the steps in your words written right here.

A major goal of the training is for the child to internalize the self-instructions so that he/she is able to use them to think slowly through potential solutions to problems that occur outside therapy. Toward this end, the therapist works to aid the child to use the self-instructions privately. Thus, use of the self-instructions by both the therapist and the child fades from overt (out loud), through a whispering phase, and finally to covert (silent) speech. The shift to private speech takes place after the child has had sufficient practice with saying the steps out loud. This sequence is described in Table 5.2, and the transition from speaking in a regular voice to speaking more privately is illustrated in the following transcript.

TABLE 5.2. Sequence of Fading Self-Instructions

1. The therapist models task performance and talks out loud while the child observes.
2. The child performs the task, instructing him/herself out loud (after sufficient practice).
3. The therapist models task performance while whispering the self-instructions.
4. The therapist performs the task using covert self-instructions with pauses and behavioral signs of thinking (e.g., stroking beard or chin).
5. The child performs the task using the self-instructional steps privately.

Note. After Meichenbaum and Goodman (1971); Kendall (1977).

Therapist: OK, you try this one.

Child: Let's see, what am I supposed to do? *(Pause)* Which is more? *(Pause)* Look at all the possibilities. And you get to look at all of them carefully. I think this one *(child points to answer)*.

T: Yep, I think that's the right answer.

C: I did a good job.

T: OK, why don't you go ahead and do the next one.

C: Let's see what you're supposed to do on this one. OK, which one is less. *(Pause)* Go over all the choices. *(Pause)* I'll go over the problem again. *(Pause)* OK, I think it's the second one.

T: *(Checks the answer)*

C: I did a good job.

T: Good. Do you remember the last time when I did a problem I started whispering to myself—so I wouldn't disturb other people around me?

C: Yeah.

T: So why don't you try doing that for a while. Just think the steps, and say them to yourself. Then, I'll do the next one.

C: *(Whispering)* OK, let's see what I'm supposed to do with this problem. *(Pause)* Look carefully. OK, I think the first one is more.

T: Yep, that's right. Wanna do the next one too? Remember you can use the steps privately.

C: Let's go on. *(Pause)* Look at all the possibilities. *(Whispering)* Calculate the amounts . . . *(Pause)* OK, I'm ready. It's this one.

T: Terrific, that's right.

C: I did a good job.

T: Yes you did, you took your time, you thought to yourself, and you got the right answer.

The success of teaching self-instructions to youth is linked to several factors: (1) the interpersonal style of the therapist, (2) the enhancement of the child's involvement in the sessions, (3) the developmental level of the child, (4) the use of directed discovery, and (5) practice.

Although not easy to describe in written format, the interpersonal style of the therapist contributes to the positive outcome of self-instructional training. Being willing to be playful yet organized, respectful yet allow for kidding, and task oriented without being bossy are just a few of the ways that one could begin to describe a preferred therapist. It should be kept in mind that adopting the preferred therapeutic style is not easy for some individuals, and supervision often proves to be very helpful in the process. Therapists improve with their increased experience. Indeed, in one study (Kendall et al., 1990), where the same therapists performed the intervention for 5 months for one set of children and then again for 5 months with another set of children, the effects were, in general, greater for the children whose therapists were more experienced. Supervision of these therapists would support such an interpretation of the outcomes, because the stiffness and "manual following" that was evident in the first application was much less visible in the second application. With greater experience, therapists were much more likely to use the steps in creative, off-the-cuff ways and to have what appeared to be a more fun interaction with the children.

Creating a "fun" atmosphere in the therapy session is central to the encouragement of the child's involvement in the treatment process. As mentioned earlier, letting the child reword the problem-solving steps serves to both support involvement and add to the individualized quality of the treatment. To meet the needs of specific children, the therapist can let the child develop steps that are fewer in number (there is no magic in five steps), although we encourage the therapist to ensure that self-reward and coping statements are a part of the steps. Also, the child can choose to use another cue to remind him/her to say the steps—the stop sign receives a favorable reaction from children, but other options can be used. In addition to these modifications of the process, the therapist can actively elicit the child's ideas for use as practice training tasks (e.g., personalized role-play vignettes). In this regard, it is crucial that time be spent addressing interpersonal problems that are a concern to the child, not just the dilemma that a parent or teacher identifies as problematic. The child can thus come to understand that the use of the problem-solving ideas can be a real advantage to him/her.

Regarding development, it is generally accepted that children below a certain age level are not ready for the use of external verbal behavior to inhibit actions. Indeed, a 4-year-old who hears an adult say, "Don't put the scissors in the plug," is tuned into the idea and may seek out the plug—scissors in hand. It is not that he/she is being disobedient, but rather that, at this development stage, the external verbal behavior impels the child to action. External verbal behavior and the eventual internal verbal directives can come to inhibit behavioral action, but this requires a child who is "ready." What rule of thumb can we offer? Speaking generally, after the age of 7 children should be developmentally prepared for inhibitory control.

Directed discovery is a phrase that is intended to communicate the collaborative interaction that surrounds training in self-instructions. The therapist knows where he/she is going with the training, but the child is an active participant in the journey. The child makes decisions, contributes to the development of the steps and rules, and is allowed to invoke his own ideas in the process. In addition to consensus decision making, taking a directed discovery approach involves the therapist's asking questions, rather than making statements. Keeping the "questioning" style in mind is especially important with a structured intervention such as this, for it could be, unwittingly, too easy for the therapist to dominate the sessions. Do not impose the problem-solving process on the child; carefully elicit and shape the child's use of the process that makes sense to him/her. Clearly, the end product is a child who has learned some self-directed problem-solving statements, but the road toward this end can take many directions and the child can participate in how the journey progresses.

In the world of real estate, the answer to the question, What are the three most important factors when buying a property, is "location, location, and location." In clinical child interventions, the answer might be "practice, practice, and practice." The acquisition and successful use of self-directed statements take time. It is not the case that these steps are fully learned even when the child can recite them. More practice is needed to ensure that there is some correspondence between saying the steps and doing the steps. Employing the steps with some variations (nonrigidly) and across problem types is helpful. Taking advantage of multiple modalities is helpful as well—hence the child hears the therapist use the steps, writes the steps him/herself, and reads them again when restating them. Many, many trials are required to come to develop an internal governor that can inhibit activity.

MODELING

Why was I (PCK) embarrassed to see my younger son dunk his donut in his milk? Why—because I know where he acquired this habit. You see, dunking is not genetic; nor was it requested, required, rewarded, or otherwise encouraged. He did, however, observe me dunking at the breakfast table and modeling can be a powerful force in shaping behavior.

The therapeutic use of modeling entails the exposure of a client to an individual (or individuals) who actually demonstrates the behaviors to be learned by the client. Modeling, also referred to as observational learning, has been used to produce such diverse therapeutic and educational outcomes as the elimination of behavioral deficits, the reduction of excessive fears, and the facilitation of social behavior (Bandura, 1969, 1986; Rosenthal & Bandura, 1978). In our program, the therapist serves as an active and participating model who demonstrates the processes used in problem solving. By alternating with the child task by task, the therapist demonstrates or models problem solving and the use of the self-directed self-instructions. The cognitive-behavioral approach, therefore, involves teaching via modeling with a modicum of direct orders. The therapist does not so much tell the child what to do as work with the child showing him/her one valuable way to think through problems.

There are different ways that a model can demonstrate behavior. Some of the formats include graduated modeling, symbolic modeling, filmed modeling, and participant modeling. Perhaps the single most important distinction concerns whether the model displays "mastery" or "coping" behavior. A mastery model demonstrates ideal behavior. For instance, the mastery model demonstrates rapid and correct performance with an absence of difficulty and frustration. While this may, at first blush, seem to be the best approach, it is possible for the observer to undermine such "mastery" by thinking, for example, "Oh, it's easy for you, but I can't do it."

In contrast to the mastery model, the coping model occasionally makes mistakes and shares with the child any difficulties that are encountered while completing the tasks. The coping model demonstrates coping strategies for dealing with difficulties or failures. Thus, the coping model is more like the child than the mastery model, provides a more strategic approach, and offers methods for dealing with frustration and failure. The coping model is demonstrating performance that is more like the child's, more real, and less likely to be dismissed. Indeed, what the impulsive child needs to witness is not someone else who can do things well, but rather someone who is willing to go through the task and its steps slowly, with illustrations of how to correct errors along the way. The coping model shows how to deal with errors and frustration and also demonstrates how to, in the end, solve the problem. In terms of effectiveness, a coping model has been found to be superior to a mastery model (e.g., Kazdin, 1974; Meichenbaum, 1971; Sarason, 1975).

It is also important to note that a model who verbalizes out loud is superior to one who does not verbalize. That is, talking out loud while modeling offers a demonstration of the thinking through of a problem to a problem solution. Thus, the child is exposed to a problem solver who goes public with his/her private thoughts and displays the thinking that is behind the solution and the action. This type of exposure and practice is most potent. Meichenbaum (1971) provided data to support the statement that the most effective modeling strategy includes the model's stating out loud cognitive coping strategies.

At times, such as in early treatment sessions, the therapist performs the task correctly and focuses directly on modeling the use of the problem-solving steps. Later, and throughout the rest of training, the therapist more often serves as a coping model. This modeling takes place in relation to not only the tasks and training materials but also the therapist's routines. That is, taking advantage of the regularly occurring problems that face the therapist in his/her day, the therapist can demonstrate how he/she goes about problem solving. A lost key, an unreturned telephone call, a last-minute schedule change: All of these, and many other events, can serve to allow the therapist to be a verbalizing, coping model.

We now offer several illustrations of coping model. First, a transcript will illustrate modeling the problem-solving steps (described in more detail previously under the section of Self-Instructional Training). Next, we illustrate the therapist as a coping model on training tasks, and last, we illustrate the role of the coping model as part of routine therapeutic practice. In this sample, the task is following directions (session 2 from the *Stop and Think Workbook* [note: the second edition of the workbook contains added tasks, with some being cognitively less demanding for the children].

Therapist: OK, now we're going to use the steps [self-instructions] when we do the problems.

Child: OK.

T: The first time I'll do a couple of problems. Then you can do some. We'll sort of take turns. OK?

C: OK.

T: So, here's the problem: "Cross out everything that is not a circle. Now, put a happy face on the shape that is not crossed out." . . . What am I supposed to do here? Well, I'm supposed to do two things. First, I have to cross out shapes, then I have to make a smile face. I'm supposed to do one at a time. OK, so what I'm supposed to do first is cross out shapes — shapes that are not circles. The next step is to look at all the possibilities. So, I will look at each shape, one at a time, and decide if it's a circle. Remember, when we do problems like this one we have to pay close attention to the instructions.

C: OK, but you can't look at any answers.

T: That's right. There aren't any answers to look at. So we have to make the answer by crossing out the shapes.

C: That's an easy one!

T: So now I'll do the next step — focus in — and try to solve the problem. There, all the shapes are crossed out.

C: Um huh.

T: But wait, there was more to do . . . there was the smile face. Let's see what were the directions? Oh yes, draw a smile face in the shape that wasn't crossed out: that would be this circle. So then I must have done a good job. Let's try the next one. "If the shape is a circle, put an 'X' in it." Let's find out what I'm supposed to do this time. I'm supposed to put an "X" in the shape if it is a circle.

C: "X" the circles.

T: Yeah! That's it. OK, now focus in and just think of this problem. That's a circle so I make an "X." That's not a circle, so I pass it over. Did I do it right?

C: Yep.

T: I did it right. I took my time and I did a good job. OK, why don't you do a couple of them just like I did.

C: OK. "If the shape is white and a circle, put an 'X' in it."

T: OK.

C: Find out what I'm supposed to do.

T: Uh-huh.

C: Yeah, put an "X" in the white circles. Step 2. Um, look at the shapes and focus in. Then make the "X"s.

T: Make the "X"s?

C: Yeah, look at each one and then, if its white and, um, a circle, make an "X." *(Pause)* OK.

T: OK, let's check it out. Oh good, that's correct.

C: I did a good job.

T: You sure did.

With a minimum of direct commands, the therapist was able to get the child to use the problem-solving steps while working on the "following directions" tasks. Modeling was the key strategy. In the next transcript, which follows from the one above, the therapist serves as the *coping* model:

Therapist: I'll try the next one.

Child: OK.

T: What's the first thing we're going to do? Let's read the instructions and find out the problem. "If the shape is a square, and it has diagonal stripes, cross it out."

C: Square with stripes.

T: OK, now what? *(Pause)* Gee, it's not just the shape . . . I gotta check the lines too. Some of the other problems have been so easy I could have just written the answer; now I've really got to think.

C: Write it down on paper.

T: OK, but then what?

C: Check each one.

T: Yeah, but I'm not sure exactly. *(Pause)* Why do I have to do this one? Wait. *(Pause)* OK, I can write down square and diagonal stripes—the stripes go at an angle. Not up and down, and not straight across.

C: The first one is one, so cross it out.

T: Let me think. It's cross it out, not put an "X" inside. The shape is a square, and the lines are diagonal. So, I cross it out.

C: Yeah.

T: Now I think I've got it.

C: Yeah.

T: I almost muffed that one. But I caught myself before I gave up. I did a good job.

By serving as a coping model, the therapist demonstrates not only the use of the self-instructional problem-solving steps in the performance of the task, but also the use of coping strategies when problem solutions are not readily available. Since it is inevitable that the child will run into problems that are not readily solvable, having coping responses available will reduce the likelihood that the child will throw up his/her arms and quit, or turn against the environment and act out. Coping statements are built into the self-instructions for use after the incorrect response and are designed to replace overly negative self-statements such as, "I'm dumb" with more acceptable statements such as, "I'll have to be more careful."

The last of our transcripts in this section exhibits the use of coping modeling in the therapist's routine. Recall that we are not telling the children what to do but showing them one way to work out solutions. The tasks provide opportunities for many learning trials, but the therapist's routine activities provide additional, and possibly more potent, examples. Numerous examples come to mind, but the following "briefcase" and "room key and chairs" illustrations will suffice.

Each of us has a briefcase or purse. In either case, it is often stuffed with materials, and the beginning of each session provides the therapist with the challenge of locating the workbook and the task for that particular session. Most adults, if not all, can solve this trivial problem with ease. Nevertheless, it is a valuable opportunity for using the problem-solving steps in routine activities, thus serving as a natural coping model.

Therapist: How's your soccer team doing? *(Puts briefcase on top of desk)*

Child: Pretty good; we won our last game. I scored a goal, too.

T: Great. *(Opens briefcase upside down and some materials spill out onto the desk and floor)* Heck, why am I dumb? *(Short pause)* No, wait. I'm not dumb; I just didn't think.

C: Huh?

T: *I* didn't think. . . . I didn't remember which is the top and which is the bottom of the briefcase.

C: Oh.

T: Let's see; how can you tell which is the top? *(Examines case; child looks also)* Here, this little label is on only one side; it's on the top. If I can remember that this goes on top, then I won't spill all these things next time. *(Pause)* The label goes on top. *(Pause)* The label goes on top. *(Whispered)*

Yet another example of the therapist's serving as a cognitive coping model on routine jobs concerns finding the key to the office (therapy room) and arranging for the correct number of chairs to be in the room. We will assume that the therapist in this case uses a room other than his/her office for the individual sessions, and that this room is shared with others and has been used for other purposes. The therapist and child approach the therapy room:

Therapist: Here we are. *(Turns doorknob)* It's locked!

Child: Locked? *(Turns doorknob)*

T: Do I have the key? I don't know. Let me look in my purse. *(Opens purse, and while searching, things fall out and onto the floor)*

C: *(Laughs)*

T: Where did that key go? I always misplace it. If I could only keep it in one place. Wait, there's no hurry. No need to rush around here. I better take a look in each part of this pocketbook. First, I'll check this pocket; no, it's not there. Not here, either. Ah, here it is.

C: Can we go in now?

T: As soon as I put these things back in. *(Whispers)* Maybe I can put this key on a special hook and put it in this part of my purse. Then I'll know where it is next time. *(After entering room and getting set up)* Just a minute, Jeff. *(Goes into briefcase and removes a large paper clip)* I'll put this key here and then clip it in a special spot in my purse. Then I won't misplace it. I'll have to remember next time that I clipped it right here.

Both examples would be followed up at the next session, when, for instance, the therapist goes to open the briefcase and stops, pauses, and thinks out loud, "The label goes on top." After pausing and saying the above statement, the therapist then opens the case and says, "Good, I got the top on top—good job."

As you might suspect, the examples here are only samples and there are many instances in which routine jobs provide opportunities for coping modeling. It is desirable to use these opportunities regularly and to pause at the proper time to allow the child to provide the reminder. Experience suggests that the child will sometimes chime in, "This *(pointing)* goes on top." Such an event is a perfect opportunity to smile and provide verbal social rewards for being thoughtful.

BEHAVIORAL CONTINGENCIES

Incentive manipulation is vital, and the use of contingencies, in our opinion, is an essential feature of the training. Without rewards for learning the skills, children may be too easily pulled toward other rewarding activities. Recall, for a moment, that we define our program as an effort to maintain the demonstrated efficacies of behavioral therapy, but with the inclusion of cognitive training. Our therapy is not solely cognitive, and effective implementations are those that pay close attention to the reward system that is in effect during the learning and maintenance of the training.

The behavioral contingency features of the cognitive-behavioral therapy for impulsive children include (1) self-reward and social reward, (2) response-cost, (3) self-evaluation, (4) rewarded homework assignments ("show that I can" [STIC] tasks), and (5) rewards at termination.

Creating a Rewarding Social Context: Self-Reward and Social Reward

Behavioral contingencies typically concern dispensing rewards for desired actions. This principle—the "law of effect"—is so well established that, indeed, it truly earns the label "law." Programs for teaching children benefit from a healthy dose of reward contingencies. Two types of rewards that are employed—systematically and generously—are self-reward and social reward. Recall here that one of the self-instructions taught to the child is, "I did a good job." The exact wording does not concern us as much as the need for self-reward following successful task performance. As a part of the self-instructions that are rehearsed for each task, the child pauses to provide and profit from self-rewards.

In addition to self-reward as part of the self-instructions, we encourage therapists to foster self-reward in any instance where it would be appropriate. The increased use of self-rewards will likely enhance the child's sense of self-efficacy and positive self-esteem. For many children, their environment offers all too few opportunities for rewards, and to the extent that the therapist–child relationship can allow and aid self-reward the child will benefit.

Social reward ties in directly with the suggestion to create a rewarding environment. The therapist uses smiles, comments such as "good," "fine," and "nice job," and any of the generally socially rewarding messages appropriate with children (e.g., "all right"). These rewards set the tone of the sessions: positive, rewarding, and encouraging. Interestingly, in an analysis of therapists' verbal behavior in sessions, Braswell et al. (1985) found that statements of encouragement ("Keep up the good work," "I can see you're really trying hard," etc.) but not simple confirming statements ("That's correct," "Right," "Uh-huh," etc.) were associated with more positive child outcomes. These results are not surprising, but they do reaffirm and underscore the need for the therapeutic experience to be a rewarding one.

Rewards (prizes) are chosen with the specific individual child in mind and values are assigned to the different rewards. Making the reward menu, like the training program itself, is a collaborative give-and-take experience. Ideas are solicited from the child and included in the menu. For example, a small reward might be a National Football League pencil, a small toy could be a medium reward, with a T-shirt, Nerf ball, or cassette tape being a major reward. It seems that each child suggests one or two rewards that are so expensive or out of reach that therapist has to set some boundaries. This too is part of the process of social problem solving. Opportunities to earn rewards are available at each session, or the child can save up his earnings and work toward a major goal.

Response-Cost: Reminders to Stop and Think

A response-cost contingency operates whereby a child is given in advance a number of reward tokens (chips) and is informed that he/she can lose one for various reasons. Some of the reasons for enacting a response-cost include making a mistake on task instructions, answering the task question incorrectly, forgetting one of the self-instructions, misusing the self-instructions, and going too fast. In this way, response-cost is designed to cue the child to remember to stop and think before responding: It is a potent contingency, but it is not the only contingency and it is not to be construed as punitive. Rather, taking the chip away, with an explanation of why, cues the child about how to improve behavior and performance next time.

In the *Stop and Think Workbook* we use 20 Stop and Think dollars that the child cuts out from the hard pages at the back of the workbook. These

20 Stop and Think dollars are given to the child at the start of each session and they are his/hers to keep and use for rewards from the menu. A bank is provided in the back of the workbook, and the child and therapist keep a record of the number of Stop and Think dollars that remain at the end of each session.

Because response-cost can be misperceived as a punitive prescription, we think it worthwhile to consider the rationale for the inclusion of response-cost. Impulsive children tend to respond quickly without or before carefully evaluating all possible alternative solutions to problems; consequently, they make many mistakes. When presented with a choice of alternative answers, impulsive children will sometimes answer correctly, conceivably obtaining the right answer by chance or because the problem was so easy that the answer was immediately apparent. If one *only* reinforces an impulsive child for right answers, which can be a matter of luck or fast guessing, one in effect spuriously rewards the child for being quick and less than fully thoughtful. In order to circumvent this problem, the cognitive-behavioral strategy uses a response-cost contingency.

The following scenario from a typical classroom demonstrates why the response-cost component carries clout. The scene is a fourth-grade classroom, 26 children, one teacher, and an arithmetic lesson. The teacher asks a question during a math drill, "What is 96 divided by 12?" Hands go up almost immediately. Children excitedly wait to be called on while others call out. One impulsive child cries, "Six." A few classmates put their hands down. The child calls out again, "It's 9, the answer is 9—oh, no, it's 8, 8 times 12 is 96." The teacher, perhaps seeking no more than a renewed calm, says, "Yes, correct." The reward contingency was applied for the correct answer, but it inadvertently rewarded the fast guessing.

Now, let's rerun the scene with a response-cost procedure. Everything would proceed the same way until the child cried out, "Six." At this point, the teacher would say, "No, you're going too fast and not thinking. You lose one chip. Try to think and be sure before you answer." After a pause, the teacher asks, "OK, what is 96 divided by 12?" The child pauses and then says, "Eight." The teacher provides social praise: "Good, that's the way. Take your time and be sure you've got it right." For other examples of classroom applications, the reader is referred to Kendall and Bartel's *Teaching Problem Solving: A Manual for Teachers* (1990).

It is conceivable that a reward contingency could be arranged so that reward is given only if the child's first answer is correct. That is, after one response, other answers would not earn a reward. Theoretically, this procedure prevents the unwanted spurious rewarding of fast guessing. However, when a child does get the answer correct, the peer group may provide the rewards and the child receives some sense of accomplishment for a correct response. Thus, even if the teacher withholds reinforcement from all responses but the first one, other children and/or the child's personal perception can nevertheless provide the reward. In addition, the response-cost procedure provides a valuable cue for the child and it is accompanied by an explanation for the response-cost. These features carry with them the potential to inhibit responding.

Self-Evaluation

When behavioral contingencies are consistently and appropriately employed, the child will learn the desired behaviors. But what happens when the child leaves the environment in which the contingencies are applied, after the training is completed? As we know, the behavior is often not maintained. Self-evaluation is a strategy intended to foster maintenance.

Self-evaluation skills can be taught through the use of a "How Did You Do Today?" chart, an example taken from the *Stop and Think Workbook* is shown below:

	How Did You Do Today?				
Your rating:	1	2	3	4	5
	Not so hot	OK	Good	Very good	Super
Therapist's rating:	1	2	3	4	5

Do the ratings agree (within one point)?
If they do, you get 2 points!

The self-evaluation chart is used first by the therapist and subsequently by both the child and the therapist. For instance, at the conclusion of the second session, the therapist rates the child's performance, providing detailed feedback on how the child did for the day. This feedback includes a thorough explanation as to why the particular rating was chosen. For example, the therapist might tell the child, "You did pretty good today; you did the problems carefully and made very few mistakes. You also remembered the self-instructions. I think I would rate your performance a 4—'very good.' If you had made many errors, gone too fast, or forgotten the steps, I would probably rate you a 1—'not so good.' If you had done even better than today, by not making any mistakes at all, I probably would rate you a 5—'super extra special.'" In later sessions the child is also asked to evaluate his/her own performance, and if the child's and therapist's ratings match (exactly or within one point), the child earns additional rewards. In actual sessions, the therapist holds a sheet of paper above the center of the "How Did You Do Today?" chart so that both the child and therapist can consider the child's performance, complete the chart, and do so simultaneously but without one person seeing the other's ratings. On the transcript that follows, the interaction of the therapist and the child exemplifies the beginning of teaching self-evaluation skills.

Therapist: Here's a way you can earn two extra Stop and Think dollars. We'll use this little chart here called "How Did You Do Today?"

Child: Yeah.

T: OK, and after every session . . .

C: Yeah.

T: I select a number to describe how you did. *(Points to chart)* Underneath number 1 it says "not so good." Number 2 is "OK." Number 3 is "good." Number 4 is "very good." Number 5 is "super extra special." OK, so . . . near the end of every session, I'm going to pick a number that I think best describes how good you did. Also, I want you to pick a number to tell me how good you think you did. And if your number is the same number as mine . . .

C: Yeah.

T: Or on either side of it by just one.

C: Yeah.

T: Then I'll give you the two extra Stop and Think dollars.

C: What if it's the same?

T: If it's the same, that's terrific! It shows that you and I agreed on how well you did today and you would get the extra bonus. OK?

C: OK.

T: If you pick a rating that's just one away from the number I pick, you still get an extra chip. If your choice is more than one away from mine—very different—then you don't get a bonus. The idea is to try to be as accurate as you can in describing your behavior. Think back over our time together and recall how it went. Did you think ahead? Were you focused? How do you think you did today?

C: Ummm.

T: Think about how hard you worked, how many times I had to correct you. Then, pick a number to tell me how you think you did today.

C: Five.

T: You think you did 5?

C: Yeah.

T: I think you did very good. I think you did "very good" (4) because you got two wrong, OK, and a few times you forgot to do all the steps.

C: Yeah.

T: And sometimes you skipped ahead a little bit so you weren't "extra super special"—I gave you a "very good"—number 4. OK.

C: Now mine's a 5 and your's is a 4. Just one away.

T: So you get the bonus. It was only one away from the rating I picked.

Evaluating their behavior every 10 or 15 minutes can be effective for some extremely inattentive, impulsive children. This can be done for the first several therapy sessions, gradually increasing the evaluation interval over the course of treatment. In this way, the therapist breaks down the unit of observation to a duration that can be managed by the child. As the child's ratings of his/her behavior come to consistently match the therapist's, the unit of observation is increased. While this task of self-observation may appear to be easy to us, it isn't for ADHD children. Researchers have noted that enhancing self-observation capacities seems to be a critical need for many ADHD children. In addition, investigators from disparate research teams have demonstrated that cognitive-behavioral methods can be effective in improving the self-monitoring of such children (Hinshaw & Erhardt, 1991).

STIC Tasks: Homework Assignments

Given the high desirability of having the child practice problem solving and learning to stop and think outside as well as inside the therapy session, homework assignments are included as part of the training. But, as anyone who has ever worked with children knows, homework is not a favorite word or activity. Instead, we refer to out-of-session tasks using "STIC" tasks. Each task is an opportunity for the child to show that he/she can do something.

The STIC assignments are "graded" in two ways. First, they are graded according to acceptability—if the assignment is completed in an acceptable fashion, the child earns a bonus. Second, they are graded in terms of a hierarchy of difficulty. Early assignments are less complex and easier than later assignments. For example, at the end of the very first therapy session, the child is asked to remember the therapist's name. The STIC task is easy, but a contingency is established nonetheless: The child can earn a bonus (e.g., two Stop and Think dollars) at the start of the next session if he/she can recall the name of the therapist. In later sessions, the STIC task is more directly related to the training, such as asking the child to be able to recall all of the problem-solving steps. In later sessions, the child's STIC task involves his/her providing a description of an instance where he/she *could have used* the self-instructional steps. This task is designed simply to get the child to identify instances in which using the steps would be appropriate. In even later sessions, the child must describe an instance in which he/she *actually used* the problem-solving process in the classroom or at home. Here the emphasis is on actual deployment of self-instructions outside the specific therapy sessions. If all goes well, the child becomes accustomed to beginning each session with a discussion of the STIC task. For much of treatment, this involves the child's informing the therapist of instances outside of treatment in which being an active problem solver proved to be useful.

It is, of course, possible for the child to tell a story about using the self-instructional steps that was not in fact true. For instance, when asked how he/she used the self-instructions last week, the child might fabricate the response, "When doing my homework." Although we have no way of knowing for certain whether this is an accurate report, we reward the response since it is an instance in which the self-instructions could be quite helpful. Often, we then inquire further: "Oh, how did you use the steps when doing your homework?" If the child doesn't know or says, "Well, I really didn't," we state that it would be a good time to use self-instructions but that he/she only gets the reward when he/she actually uses the steps. We add, however, that next session will be another chance. "If you can tell me when you actually used the problem-solving steps in class or at home, you can earn the bonus, OK?" Children's responses are rapidly shaped so that they soon learn to describe how they used the steps. The veracity of the event cannot be checked so we reward the child for providing an apt description of when to use the steps.

Therapist: Remember what we talked about at our last meeting? We agreed that you could start out today earning a bonus. You can earn it by reporting on your STIC task—for today that involves telling me how you used the self-instructions in class or at home.

Child: Yeah.

T: So, how did your STIC task go?

C: When I was arguing with my brother, I thought about another idea.

T: *(Pause)* And . . .

C: Well, it doesn't matter what he thinks cause he's little and doesn't really know. So, I just said yeah sure and went ahead. I thought that it was better than getting into a fight.

T: Did you think of any other choices?

C: No, just that one. So I thought it over and then I did it.

T: Was it OK?

C: Yeah; he stopped bothering me and we went back to playing.

T: Uh-huh; so you did it right.

C: Yeah.

T: Anything else?

C: Oh *(sheepish smile)*, then I told myself I did a good job.

T: Great job, you definitely get your bonus because you did a really good job of remembering to do the STIC task. Of course, I don't know if you actually remembered to tell yourself that you did a good job *(smile)*, but you can do that now—you did do a good job.

C: How many dollars do I have now?

For younger children, stickers can be used as a further reward for successful completion of the STIC tasks. For older children, stickers may not be necessary, but one can begin to refer to successful STIC tasks as evidence that the training has stuck. Each completion of a STIC task is an opportunity for rewarding the child, for discussing and describing additional contexts in which the problem solving has applicability, and for helping the child to make internal attributions for his/her achievements. The rehearsal of the effort of last week is an excellent opportunity to shape and encourage the child's taking personal responsibility for personal gains. After all, the child is learning some sophisticated interpersonal thinking—becoming an "aware wolf"—and deserves to have such accomplishments fully recognized.

Rewards at Termination

Reaching the end of the treatment program is an accomplishment for the child and, no matter how easily it is dismissed by the child, the therapist is encouraged to make a big deal of the gains that have been seen. Not all children show the same positive reactions, and not all children improve to the same degree, but the thrust of the situation at termination is a recounting of the progress that has been achieved. Two strategies combine to help the child see and describe these gains: (1) the certificate and (2) the "SHOW off" tape.

There are many instances in which youth complete an activity—swimming class, boy scouts, or a recreation center summer program—and in which they are given some sign of their accomplishment. Therapists can do the same, and we encourage the use of certificates of accomplishment. For example, the last page of the *Stop and Think Workbook* is a just such a certificate for use in recognizing the child's accomplishments. The certificate may be framed, tacked to the wall, or taped to the refrigerator door—no matter, as along as it serves to document for the child (and the parents or teacher) that efforts were made and gains were the result.

A specific and crucial element in maintenance and generalization begins with the final sessions of therapy. Indeed, it is at this time that the child is helped to make a "SHOW" off tape. To SHOW off is to "SHow Others hoW." Using a portable videorecorder, the child can make a tape of a poem, a rap song, a TV commercial, or any other activity that helps other children to learn how to stop and think. Of course, because this activity is potentially time-consuming (and quite fun), the therapist introduces the idea several sessions before the last one, and uses the STIC tasks to help shape up the child's ideas for the SHOW off tape. For example, the child and therapist might switch roles, with the child acting as the therapist and teaching the therapist—now child client to learn to be less impulsive. Not only does this provide the child with the chance to be in control, but it also allows the child to demonstrate what has been learned and to be excited about owning the new skills.

By giving the role of director to the child, the therapist allows the child to put a personal signature on the problem-solving process and its meaning and utility. The process helps to strengthen the vital link between simple skills and their assimilation into everyday use. The child's SHOW off tape (also sometimes referred to as a commercial for Stop and Think) is copied and given to the child. When possible, arrangements are made to show the tape to others.

We place a great deal of emphasis on the positive endorsement of the problem-solving process and the child's acquisition and use of the process in day-to-day activities. Termination of treatment should not be viewed or described as the end of the process. Rather, it is the start of the child's opportunity to try it on his/her own. If the child stumbles along the way, booster sessions, phone contacts, or other contacts can be arranged to further instill the utility of the program and its application in the child's life.

THE ROLE OF EMOTIONS: AFFECTIVE EDUCATION

There are two important roles for affect within cognitive-behavioral therapy for impulsive children. First, improving the child's ability to accurately recognize and label his/her own emotional experiences, as well as the emotions of others, may be a necessary step for improved interpersonal problem solving. Toward this end, the training program includes tasks that require the child to label the emotions associated with various facial expressions, bodily postures, or problematic interpersonal situations. Materials used to generate such discussions are provided in several sections of the *Stop and Think Workbook*.

Second, make the child aware of the nature of his/her own emotions, the association between emotions and outbursts, and the usefulness of self-controlled self-talk in the mediation of emotional reactions. Toward this end, role-play exercises are undertaken during which the child and therapist practice using self-talk to "keep cool" and think of ways to respond other than impulsive outbursts. Although the manner in which these role-play exercises are conducted is addressed in the next section, it should be noted that one reason for including role-play activities is to heighten the child's level of emotional involvement and arousal. Thus, the child has an opportunity to practice the self-instructional problem-solving skills while grappling with problematic situations that may "pull for" a more impulsive, emotional type of responding.

Clearly when a child is working one on one with a therapist, it may be difficult for his/her role plays to produce the level of affective response that might typify the same interaction if it occurred with a family member or peer. Within appropriate limits, however, the therapist should work toward such realism. When the treatment is conducted with groups of children, it may be quite possible to generate very realistic levels of emotional arousal. For example, Goodwin and Mahoney (1975) had their elementary-school-aged subjects practice displaying self-control in the face of verbal taunts by having the children play a game in which they actually called each other names. It is possible to generate affect by having children be required to give each other a compliment, to self-identify a personal weakness, or to do something that they know they are not very good at doing. When the training situation includes opportunities for utilizing self-instructions in emotionally arousing situations, one is, in effect, beginning to train for generalization.

ROLE PLAYS

Role playing, in conjunction with thinking through the problem situation, offers an opportunity to act out the behavior and provides a performance base for the intervention. Role plays can be arranged for either hypothetical situations or situations that are actually problems for the child. Typically, both types of problem situations are employed in a sequence that facilitates the child's involvement, reduces the likelihood of resistance, and enlivens the activity of treatment. Toward these ends, role plays of hypothetical problem situations best precede "real" problem situations. Sample hypothetical situations include:

> You are watching television, and your mother/sibling changes the channel.

You tear your pants at recess and someone is making fun of you.

You are having trouble with a worksheet and your friend is already finished.

You are playing a new game and your friend starts to cheat.

Each situation can be written on an index card in advance and, once the child understands what is involved in a role-play task, one index card can be selected from a deck of cards that becomes the situation for the role play. Role plays are brief (2 to 4 minutes) and are enhanced by the therapist who identifies key elements of the situation, mentions each character who is present (including his/her role, location, and feelings), and uses props when available. In short, make the role-play activities as real as possible. Situation cards with sample problem situations, as well as blank cards, are provided in the *Stop and Think Workbook*

While one or several of these "hypothetical" situations may be a real problem situation for the child, they are quite general and likely to be problems for many children so that the specific child is not likely to feel directly targeted. After the child and therapist have gained experience with the hypothetical role plays, real problem situations can be performed. One suggested way to introduce real problem situations into the session is to write the situation on a new index card and include it among the cards for which role plays will be chosen. If one or two cards among three or four choices are real problem situations, it is quite likely that at least one will be chosen. We have found teachers and parents to be valuable sources of descriptions of the problem situations for children. Via individual consultation with a child's teacher, for example, accurate and properly worded real situations for role plays can be acquired. Proper wording is important. For instance, a child is reported by the teacher as getting in trouble for "visiting," not out-of-seat behavior and not talking. "Visiting" had a special meaning, and when the child selected the card for role playing that read, "You are in class and the teacher singles you out for visiting—you get in trouble for visiting," the child knew exactly what was meant.

Once the child has become accustomed to the role-play format, each new situation can easily be acted out. Since the first few role plays may feel somewhat awkward for both the therapist and child, special attention can be paid to the transition. In an effort to overcome the initial difficulties in moving from just talking about situations to acting them out, we have found the following format to be quite helpful.

First, just as in previous sessions, the child is asked to state the problem. For example, after the child has selected one of the situation cards, the following interaction might ensue.

Therapist: OK, what does your card say?

Child: It says, "You are watching television but your little brother keeps changing the channel."

T: So what is your problem? Or, to use your "step words," what are you supposed to do?

C: Well, I guess I'm supposed to figure out how to stop him.

T: OK.

For the second problem-solving step, the child looks at the possibilities. The therapist's role at this point is to help the child understand that in social situations, the child has to generate or create his/her own possibilities for action. In our work, we typically urge the child to think of at least three or four different alternatives for coping with each situation. During this step, the emphasis is clearly on *generating* alternatives, with evaluation of the quality of each possibility being held until later. At this time the therapist–child interaction might resemble the following.

Therapist: You know what the problem is, what are some different things you can do about it?

Child: I could hit my brother, hit him hard, but then my mom would really be mad.

T: We can think about which idea will be best to do in just a moment. For now, let's just note that one possibility you thought of would be to hit your brother. What would be another choice? Let's see if you can think of at least two more possibilities.

C: Uh . . . I could tell my mom!

T: Yes, that's an idea. You could tell your mother. What's another idea?

C: I could *try* to work out a deal with my brother. Give him something to go away.

T: Good. That's three different possibilities. You could hit your brother, you could tell your mom, or you could try to work out a deal with your brother.

Continuing with problem/solving in role plays, the therapist then translates the third step—think hard or focus—into the process of evaluating the relative merits of each alternative. We recommend attempting to evaluate the possibilities in terms of their behavioral and emotional consequences for the child and for the other people involved in the situation. Asking what might happen addresses the behavioral consequences, whereas asking how each character would feel addresses the emotional consequences. Such an evaluation process might resemble the following interchange.

Therapist: All right. You've thought of three different choices or possibilities. Now let's focus in and think hard about each one. What might happen if you decided to hit your little brother?

Child: Well, he'd get mad and start crying. Then he'd probably go tell mom and I'd get in trouble.

T: Would hitting your brother mean you would get to watch your TV program?

C: No. I'd probably get sent to my room.

T: And how would people feel after you hit your brother?

C: Well, my brother and mother would be mad. It might feel good to hit my brother (*pause*), but it wouldn't feel good to have to go to my room.

T: Let's think about the next choice—telling your mom. What might happen if you did that?

C: Well, my brother would probably get mad, but if mom took my side, I might get to watch my show. Of course, mom doesn't really like it when we tattle on each other.

T: So that choice has some good things about it and some bad things. What about the last one?

C: What was it? . . . Oh, yeah, try to work out a deal with my brother. I don't know, but maybe my brother and I could decide that I get to keep watching my show but he could pick what we watch next. Then he'd be happy and I'd be happy and mom wouldn't know anything about it.

T: OK. You've done some careful thinking about your three choices.

The next problem-solving step involves picking an answer. With social problems, there is often more than one good answer or good way to solve a problem. With more cognitively sophisticated children, the therapist may also wish to add that in other, more difficult situations, none of the choices may seem very good and in those cases one has to try to pick the "least bad" solution. With regard to the child's actual choice, if the therapist is satisfied that the child has participated in problem solving, generated several alternatives, and evaluated each possibility, the actual response the child selects is of *less* importance. To use the current example, if, after examining the consequences, the child decides that it still might be worth it to hit his/her little brother, the child is allowed to select this choice without receiving a response-cost. After all, it is the thinking process that we are teaching—not what to think but how to think. The therapist should feel free to state why he/she thinks another alternative would be more optimal—has fewer unwanted, negative consequences—but the child's choice should be respected.

The self-reward step can be handled much as it is with impersonal problem-solving tasks. The child is encouraged to use a self-reinforcing statement to reward his/her good problem solving. Coping statements are also used as part of the social problem-solving process.

Once a reasonably clear understanding of how the steps can be used to solve social problems has been developed, one need not rigidly adhere to the exact steps that were used in the earlier sessions. The following transcript contains a description of the therapist and child working or defining the role-play task and then using the steps in a more informal manner. In this case, the therapist and child talk about the problem and then act it out.

Therapist: You want to call your friend Sam, but your mom is on the phone. OK. Do you need to think to figure that one out?

Child: Yeah. What are we supposed to do with these problems? Act them out?

T: OK, yeah, we'll act out this one.

C: You know about this; just say, "Get off the phone."

T: OK, but then what would happen?

C: Trouble.

T: Probably.

C: Could ask her to get off.

T: What would be the consequences of that?

C: Huh?

T: What would be the consequences of asking her to get off? That means, what would happen then?

C: I don't know.

T: Would your mom get off the phone if you asked her to get off? *(Child nods yes)* Would she? That's a good possibility then.

C: I could just walk over to Sam's house.

T: That's a possibility.

After the therapist and child have become accustomed to role plays, problems that are specific to the child are introduced as the content of the role plays, the response-cost contingency is applied to errors, and so on. The therapist begins to expect generally more thoughtful and successful behaviors within the role plays and uses the contingencies to shape such improvement.

It is important for the therapist to play an active role in acting out problem situations, but the child's suggestions and input regarding the setup of each role-play situation are extremely meaningful. The therapist would be wise to encourage the child's participation by getting the child to fill in the details of the problem situation (Where is it happening? Who else is there? What are they doing?). The therapist can also get the child's feedback about aspects of the dialogue (Would your mom really say that like I just did? What would she say?).

Some children may become quite excitable during role playing. An increase in emotional arousal is actually quite desirable; however, this arousal may occasionally take the form of giddiness or silliness that actually impedes the conduct of meaningful role plays. At such times, or at any other point at which the child's behavior appears to be somewhat out of control, the therapist could hold up the stop sign (the one that has served as the cue card during the early training sessions) or ask the child to "freeze" as though he/she were a statue. After capturing the child's attention in this manner, the therapist can focus attention on the child's current behavior and ask the child to problem-solve about what other ways he/she might handle the present ongoing situation.

Our experience suggests that if the therapist initiates the role plays with enthusiasm and a willingness to share his/her own awkwardness about having to "be an actor" with the child, these sessions can be an involving and enjoyable learning experience for the child. Stated differently, the therapist can use the initiation of the role playing as yet another opportunity to be a coping model. The demonstration videotape available from the first author includes several examples of role-play interactions.

TRAINING TASKS

While we cannot overemphasize the fact that the actual tasks used in training are not as important relative to the *method* or *thinking process* that is being taught, we would like to describe those aspects of the nature and sequence of the tasks that do appear to contribute to the effectiveness of training. We also describe, briefly, features of the aforementioned *Stop and Think Workbook* as an illustration of an appropriate sequence of training tasks. Finally, we mention some ideas for extending the intervention when needed.

We recommend a progression from impersonal, cognitive tasks to more interpersonal, emotionally laden material. Beginning with simple tasks allows the child to devote more attention to the new self-instructional problem-solving process without becoming bogged down in personal problems. The *Stop and Think Workbook*, for example, begins with a simple task ("which one comes next?"), which most children find totally nonthreatening. Other tasks such as "following directions" are emphasized in subsequent sessions. In this edition, a wider range of tasks are made available for the therapist to use—thus allowing a better match between the task's demands and the child's cognitive capabilities.

Later sessions employ games that provide a transition between psychoeducational problems and more socially oriented games. We have found that children respond well to word search games where the players have to focus in (the *Stop and Think Workbook* provides a cutout drawing of a magnifying glass to use for focusing). Tangram puzzles are an example of a pattern-matching task that combines elements of a cognitive problem and a game.

Next, we introduce more typical games, such as checkers. This allows the child to practice the application of the steps with more common activities. The game-type interaction also provides an opportunity for the therapist to begin asking the child more about the types of situations that are most troublesome. A new game, Cat and Mouse, can be introduced. Applying the steps with a totally new game provides an interesting opportunity for transfer of the self-instructional skills for both the therapist and the child.

We recognize that it is helpful for the child to bring in real samples of schoolwork and we recommend that the child practice using self-instructional skills with these assignments. For example, the child and therapist can collaborate to assist the child in applying the problem-solving steps in completing math worksheets, developing a strategy for studying for a test, or when working on written assignments. Using a problem-solving approach to help the child develop a step-by-step approach to a complex task (social studies or science project) can also be a valuable learning experience.

Later in the program, the material becomes more relevant to interpersonal problem solving, because it focuses on the accurate recognition and labeling of emotions. This allows the child to think about the role of emotion in his/her behavioral responses and the types of emotions produced in various interpersonal situations. The discussion of interpersonal situations goes even further by asking the child to think of alternative responses in problematic situations and the possible emotional and behavioral consequences of each alternative. Finally, in many of the later sessions, the child is assisted in role playing the various alternatives for problematic situations, with the primary focus being on situations that are particularly difficult for that child.

A GOAL: BUILDING A COPING TEMPLATE

Cognitive-behavioral theorists have promoted the notion that individuals perceive and make sense of the world and their experiences in it through their cognitive structures. These structures are also referred to as schema or templates. Such a template has an influence on what is perceived, how perceptions are processed, and what information will be remembered in the future. Impulsive children need to develop a template that includes stopping and thinking.

Optimally, the therapist is a collaborating consultant who, as guided by the child and the child–therapist interaction, directs the discovery and practice of the use of problem-solving self-talk. This directed practice involves building bridges from the child's present level of understanding to newer, more functional levels. The interaction with the therapist supports and extends the child's development, while communicating respect, interest, and enjoyment.

Our treatment builds on educational and interpersonal experiences, as well as therapist-coached reconceptualizations of problems to build a "coping" template. That is, the treatment goal is for the child to develop a new structure, or a modified existing structure, through which he/she can look at problems in a "problem-to-be-solved" fashion. The child's acquisition and use of the coping template are major goals of treatment.

CHAPTER 6

Optimizing Treatment Impact

onfidence in the chosen therapeutic strategy, enthusiasm for the
therapist–child interaction, and knowledge of the treatment program all contribute to a rewarding and effective intervention. But
even when confidence, enthusiasm, and knowledge are high, there are no
guarantees that the desired gains will be forthcoming. Indeed, monitoring
progress and adjusting the implementation of the program are necessary
to further facilitate optimal gains.

In an effort to provide guideposts that will facilitate the implementation of the cognitive-behavioral program, we describe and discuss several
factors that offer promise as means of enhancing effectiveness. Next, the
discussion turns to the pitfalls, or potential pitfalls, that can undermine the
provision of an effective intervention and suggestions on how to avoid
them. Finally, we remind the reader of the individual difference factors,
such as age and intellectual ability, that were examined earlier in this book
as possible moderators of the effectiveness of the procedures. Whether
stressing the things "to do," the things "not to do," or the features of
children with whom things "should be done," this chapter emphasizes the
various factors that contribute to an optimally effective intervention.
Because we feel that an effective program often includes collaborations
with parents and teachers, Chapter 7 ("Working with Parents, Teachers,
and Groups of Children") is also a part of our description of ways to
optimize treatment impact.

MATCHING CHILD NEEDS TO TREATMENT STRENGTHS

Assessment and selection are required for matching the type of behavioral
problem with the intervention of choice. Perhaps more than any other
suggestion for optimizing treatment gains, the careful assessment and
proper selection of children deserve special emphasis. We have already
discussed in earlier chapters both the nature of the deficit and assessment
strategies for selection and evaluation. The reemergence of these topics at
this time is nevertheless justified because of their importance.

Consider the following case. June was a 9-year-old girl referred from
a child psychiatry service in a university medical center. She had been

154

diagnosed as hyperactive and was receiving methylphenidate, but she was still reportedly getting into serious trouble at home for impulsive behavior. Her mother had reported that she was out of control and very mischievous—"She just doesn't think." At first blush, the referral seemed appropriate.

A subsequent interview with June's mother revealed that she had an idiosyncratic perspective on impulsive behavior. For instance, June's mother had decided that June could not wear jeans to school. Since the school permitted jeans and many of June's peers wore them, the no-jeans rule was a point of contention. One day June packed a pair of jeans with her school supplies and once at school changed clothes. Because June had to take her medications, she had to report to the school office routinely. On this particular day she forgot and June's mother was notified. In an effort to take action, June's mom went to pick up June from school and caught her wearing the jeans.

The incident is not uncommon among youngsters. What is uncommon, however, is the perception of this type of rule breaking as impulsive. June planned to wear the jeans, arranged to have a way to get them to school, and was planning a change of clothes before going home. A great deal of forethought, planning, and scheming went into the event. Hardly an impulsive child.

As it turned out, June's "problems" were largely related to her mother's personality and her mother's sense of ambivalence about the child. With regard to personality, the mother was a rigid, absolutistic, and perfectionistic woman. She was employed part time as a proofreader and prided herself on not missing a single error. If she said no jeans, then it was to be no jeans. Never! Absolutely never. Not even for a special picnic day at school. And, when June and her mom were baking cookies, if it was to be two dozen, then it would be 24 cookies. Not 25, and not 23. When doing dishes, you did silverware first, glasses second, dishes third. That was the order.

For this woman, the fact that June was a foster child and that her "mother" was a foster mother created ambivalence: "Do I adopt her as my own? No, she's a problem child. . . . Yes, I must care for her." The verbalized ambivalence was also evident in behavior. Sometimes, "mother and daughter" were close; other times "foster mother" threatened "foster child" with being sent to an institution.

Was June an appropriate referral for cognitive-behavioral training? Apparently not, although it appeared that the mother was in need of an intervention to alter her belief system and its unwanted impact on those around her. Without careful assessment and selection, June might have been an unsuccessful case, causing frustration for parent and child and perhaps (mistakenly) leading the therapist to conclude that the procedures were ineffective. Forethought and planning on the part of the interviewer, in the form of assessment and selection, cannot be ignored.

Adam was an 11-year-old boy who was diagnosed as ADHD. He was receiving medication and was attending a special school. His teachers commented that he did not seem to have friends—he played team sports and often pushed his way into the crowd, but he was never sought after as a pal and was without a close friend. Reports from teachers and parents were consistent: Adam interrupted others, butted into activities, blurted out in class, demanded his way, tantrummed when rejected, and, on occasion, showed impulsive acting out and yelling. His interpersonal behavior was quite impulsive, as was his academic work. His parent and teacher ratings were consistent with his diagnosis as hyperactive, his SCRS score was 174 (>160, <200), his IQ was in the normal range, his parents were cooperative and supportive, and his teachers were willing to go along with occasional classroom monitoring of his efforts at problem solving. Adam began treatment without hesitancy—as usual, he jumped right in.

After completing 20 sessions, Adam had amassed a new set of skills. He had worked through the *Stop and Think Workbook* (Kendall, 1992a), earned prizes and a certificate, knew the problem-solving steps by heart, could discuss their use in impersonal and social contexts, and had made several "individualized" uses of the self-control process. For instance, he learned quickly that when playing games (e.g., cards) it is usually the case that you play "dealer's choice." This notion, which carried interpersonal meaning for Adam, helped him to realize and accept that taking turns was an important part of making and keeping friends. His favorite "step" was the self-statement "dealer's choice"—no one else knew what it meant exactly, and Adam relished in his special status. Adam was able to monitor himself in interpersonal activities just as he had practiced during therapy.

Adam very much enjoyed being a detective—looking for clues in social situations and using them to decide how to behave. It was Adam who suggested that, as a practice exercise, we walk through the neighborhood and look for clues about who had been there, what had gone on, or what was likely to happen in the future. Time spent in this activity was rewarding for Adam, as well as an opportunity to practice using problem-solving steps to make decisions.

An incident at summer camp was appropriately labeled a relapse, and several booster sessions were undertaken. Indeed, there has been additional contact since termination, and new problems are cast into the problem-solving mode. Progress has been maintained, although it is the therapist's suspicion that less parental infringement on the child's own thinking and decision making would, in the long run, be more beneficial.

Although one cannot be absolutely certain in an anecdotal case study such as this is, there was specific evidence and it was the therapist's impression that Adam learned the utility of self-directed speech in interpersonal contexts and that he benefited greatly from the process of acquiring self-control skills. A successful sleepover at a friend's home, bike trips with classmates, and an overall improved school performance led those involved to report noticeable improvements.

The two cases that we have described are illustrations of good and not-so-good matches between the nature of the child's difficulties and the strengths of the treatment strategy. The outcomes reflect the merits of the program when applied in a properly defined case. Though we will not go into additional detailed examples, there is a "good match" when the child displays impulsivity, lacks problem-solving skills, fails to recognize interpersonal cues, or otherwise acts without thinking. These matches hold whether or not the child is diagnosed as ADHD, Conduct Disorder, ODD, or learning disabled, for there are impulsive features in each of these behavioral problem areas.

The child is not a good candidate for cognitive-behavioral therapy *for impulsivity* if the major referral problem is depression and/or anxiety. The nature of the cognitive problem seen in impulsive youth is a deficiency in thinking, and the present treatment teaches the needed thinking skills. The nature of the cognitive disorder in depression and anxiety is linked more to a distorted manner of information processing (as opposed to a deficiency) and therefore requires an intervention that targets changing the existing maladaptive thinking pattern (Kendall, 1990; Kendall, Chansky, et al., 1992).

There are numerous instances when the treatment of choice is actually a combination of interventions. For instance, an extremely high score on the SCRS (e.g., >200) indicates that the child has problems greater than a simple deficit in self-control. Interventions that can and have been combined include medication and cognitive-behavioral therapy, cognitive-behavioral treatment for the child and parents separately, and the use of cognitive-behavioral procedures with the family (see Braswell & Bloomquist, 1991). Other combinations are appropriate as well, and we encourage readers to make the appropriate integrations.

COOPERATION AND COLLABORATION

Children are not known for their willingness to cooperate with adults. When the presence of adults is imposed on the child, as opposed to being self-selected, relationship difficulties can be exacerbated and it is not uncommon for certain teachers, coaches, or therapists to have difficulties interacting with children—especially behavioral problem children. An effective therapeutic relationship must overcome these inherent drawbacks and the therapist must make a conscious effort to achieve cooperation and collaboration.

Regarding cognitive-behavioral training, we cannot emphasize enough the need to work toward and with collaboration. That is, both the end goal and the process require the therapist and child to work together. For example, the therapist and the child take turns when rehearsing the self-instructional steps. Turn taking not only enhances the relationship and friendship between therapist and child but also requires collaboration. Collaborating in the initial sessions, even if it as elementary as passing the *Stop and Think Workbook* back and forth, sets the foundation for collaboration during later sessions involving more complicated and sophisticated problems.

Role playing the resolution to problem situations requires collaboration. Therapist and child have to work together to determine the roles to be played, how the scene will be set, what problem solutions will be role-played, and what if any props will be used. It is this decision-making process that requires collaboration, for without it the therapist would be merely dictating the paces through which the child should step. As we know, the child's involvement in the therapeutic process contributes to the achievement of desired gains (Braswell et al., 1985) and the therapist must encourage collaboration as a part of involving the child in the treatment process. In role plays, asking the child, "What do you think" and following through on some of the suggestions is one concrete method of involving the child. Similarly, recognizing when the child is involved, such as when a suggestion is offered, and rewarding him/her must be a part of the therapist's awareness throughout the program.

Cooperation and collaboration also refer to enlisting the support of significant others in the child's environment. Teachers and parents come to mind first since they often create and control the environments in which children spend most of their time, and in the following chapter we describe some strategies for working with these important groups.

ADDRESSING RELAPSE

Select setbacks are a part of the process of learning a new behavioral pattern. Indeed, the setbacks, as well as advances, are to be expected as a normal part of learning. Given the inevitability of setbacks or a resurgence of a problem situation in which the trained skills were inappropriately applied, forgotten, or ineffective, paying direct attention to the management of setbacks is encouraged. We are recommending, not unlike what Marlatt (1979) has encouraged in the treatment of alcohol problems, that a part of the initial remedial intervention address the methods and skills and the desired cognitive interpretations for overcoming the inevitable relapse and failure experiences.

By setting the expectation that "things happen," the therapist opens the door and pays attention to setbacks and partial failures. Brownell, Marlatt, Lichenstein, and Wilson (1986) differentiated between the terms *lapse* and *relapse*. A lapse refers to a process, such as a behavioral slip, that may or may not portend a negative outcome. A negative outcome would be a relapse. For example, certain aspects or applications of the problem-solving process may be forgotten, inappropriately or ineffectively applied, or even undermined by others despite the child's best efforts. Left unchecked, a temporary lapse such as this can lead children to question their ability to use the new thinking skills or to question the merits of the problem-solving steps. The risk of relapse increases as the child may abandon further use of problem solving. The intervention has to deal with the unwanted potential effects of unchecked partial failures. On the other hand, proactive efforts that directly address the inevitability of slips or mistakes (lapses) greatly reduce the likelihood of relapse (and possible collapse). Importantly, to prevent parental misperceptions from undermining treatment, parents must be informed that a lapse is not the same as a collapse. To make maximum therapeutic use of treatment lapses, the therapist should address two aspects of the situation: (1) the potential emotional setback associated with mistakes and (2) the important information communicated by the circumstances of the relapse.

Addressing the Emotional Impact of Lapses

Assume for the moment that child and therapist have progressed approximately three-quarters of the way through the program and that, until now, the child has succeeded in learning the problem-solving steps, controlling impulsive behavior, and implementing the skills in the classroom context. Assume also that the child is now involved in the school carnival and that he/she has $3 to spend on the various activities. Starting at one booth, he/she spends $2.75 and, when seeing a later, more appealing booth, is short of funds for other activities. The child thinks:

> I'm out of money; where can I get more. Oh, no one will give me their money cause they want it. Darn it, I wanted to try shooting baskets [game at the booth]. Heck. *(Pause)* I guess I should have saved some money or maybe not spent so much on the water pistol game. If I'd only thought to look at all the booths first. I'm an idiot. I'll never learn to stop and think.

Left uncorrected, this type of thinking can leave marked negative effects. First, the child is making an internal and global attribution for his/her failure. Second, the child is abandoning hope. Third, the child has discounted the merits of the problem-solving program—not by saying it doesn't or can't work, but by saying he/she can't do it. The entire monologue depicts a loss of self-confidence, a drop in self-efficacy and self-mastery, and a "why not give up" attitude.

Addressing relapse involves the specific targeting of failure experiences as part of the initial training program. During the training, the child routinely makes some errors, as does the therapist. The "handling" of these error experiences provides the basis for the therapist's assisting the child to manage failure. Therapist modeling, particularly the coping and verbalizing form of modeling, serves to initiate relapse training. The following examples illustrate the procedure during different stages of the program.

Any of the initial sessions provide opportunities for the therapist to model coping with failures—such as a failure to recall the separate self-instructional steps. As part of the self-instructional steps, the child is taught to use a coping statement after an error. This, too, is a prompt for the therapist to remember to address relapse. For instance (after the child makes a mistake):

Therapist: Oh, was that one too difficult? Maybe. But he did go too fast and that may have been the reason. I know he can do better when he takes his time. We have to practice going slower.

The therapist is sure to make errors him/herself and to be a coping and verbalizing model in response to these errors. While doing some of the activities in the workbook, it is likely that both child and therapist will have some unsuccessful experiences (e.g., giving a wrong answer, not thinking of an alternative solution). If, as in one of the games, the contest is close and the child is truly trying to win, a setback can seriously undermine the progress that has been made. Such occurrences, nevertheless, provide opportunities for the therapist to address the fact that they are chance occurrences and not due to anything the child might have done or said. Parts of some games are skill—and one can work to improve these parts, but other parts are chance and no one can control chance. When it is the therapist's turn and something negative results from chance, the therapist might think aloud:

Heck, that sets me back a lot. You're gonna win. Darn. I was trying hard too! (Pause) Well, all I can do is answer the questions—I can't control the roll of the dice. That wasn't my fault, it was just bad luck. (Pause) I'll keep trying, so when my luck is good I can maybe win the game.

Both the STIC tasks (homework assignments) and the role-play exercises provide opportunities to address relapse. In fact, it is in these contexts that the notion of relapse training is dealt with most directly.

Therapist: Do you remember last time we met I said you could earn some extra chips if you could tell me about a time when you used the steps? Can you tell me a time?

Child: No, I forgot.

T: Oh, well. Let's take some time now and try to think.

C: I can't think of anything.

T: Last week you told me about how you used the steps to think about making your lunch for the bike ride. That was a terrific example. This week you don't have one, but maybe next week you will. I'll remind you at the end of today's meeting. You did well last time so I'm sure you can do it again. This one time doesn't mean you can't do it later on. For now, let's describe a "made-up" experience, just so we get to practice thinking it through.

It is often the case that a "superhero" can be used as a coping example—a model of how to bounce back after a temporary setback. Certainly, many sports figures (from all of the sports) have temporary slumps in their performance. Characters such as Superman, Batman, Spiderman, or a Teenage Mutant Ninja Turtle can serve as a superhero model. Once the child's superhero is identified, the therapist can later ask, "How might _____ handle this situation?" Seeing how an identified hero figure manages a difficult situation can help spark additional ideas for the child. In a group run by one of the authors, local sports heros were asked (and they responded) what they did and what they said to themselves when handling frustrating situations.

A common point of breakdown in the problem-solving process occurs when a child becomes too emotionally upset to be effective in addressing the problem situation. We suggest that it be pointed out that both others and ourselves can be obstacles to problem solving. When we are our own obstacle it is often because we are too excited, angry, or upset. Discussing a recent experience of the child, and mentioning how overreaction can interfere, can serve to open this issue for consideration. Overreacting to a parental reprimand can result in the child's being in more trouble than he was in in the first place. Even children who cannot admit to such a circumstance happening to them can usually share an example involving a sibling or classmate. Discuss how, at such moments, it is difficult for people to do their best problem solving, but they can think about these tough situations ahead of time and make a specific plan for how they want to handle themselves at such times. For example, many children benefit from planning how to escape from a situation that is disturbing so they can begin to calm down. This plan includes identifying a place to go and learning to use the time to think and employ relaxation strategies. The therapist and child can collaborate to identify the child's cognitive, affective, and physiological cues that signal an impending outburst (e.g., thinking "It's not fair," feeling angry, experiencing a flushed face and rapid breathing). These cues, as well as cues that cooperating adults might provide, serve to remind the child to remove himself from the situation. These efforts can easily be framed as "ways to keep your cool" (Braswell & Bloomquist, 1991).

Understanding the Information Communicated by Mistakes/Difficulties

As part of training and relapse prevention, children and parents are encouraged to discuss situations in which problem-solving skills were not used or were thought to be ineffective. The therapist explains that, ultimately, more can be learned from mistakes than from successes. When an unsuccessful incident arises, the therapist helps the child to analyze the situation carefully to determine the thoughts, feelings, or actions (his/her own or others) that contributed to creating a situation in which it was difficult to be an effective problem solver.

Sometimes even minor difficulties in a session can be turned into opportunities for becoming a better problem solver (or personal detective). Experiencing difficulty with the problem-solving steps and their application to real problem behaviors can be seen in the role-play sessions. Occasionally, a child will throw up his/her hands and give up.

Child: Are we done yet? I want to go. I just can't do this stuff.

Therapist: Gee, I know you didn't do well on this one, but does the one mistake mean you can't do it at all? What do you think?

C: I don't know. I guess not.

T: Let's take a short break. You know, you've done well at this before. I wonder what is making it difficult today?

C: I don't know.

T: Hmmm ... with some other kids I've known, sometimes they feel tired and that makes it difficult to concentrate. For other kids, I've learned that they may have had something else on their mind and that made it hard to concentrate. What do you think could be making it difficult for you?

C: I think I'm tired. . .I had to get to school early today, and I was up late last night.

T: If someone is tired, what might help that person feel more energetic?

C: I don't know, maybe stand up and walk around a little. Get moving.

T: Sounds like a good idea to me. Let's try it and see.

(One minute later)

T: OK, let's try another one [referring to role plays]. You know we did several of these very well before we got stuck. Let's try to do several more. Problems come up, and that's OK because we know how to solve them.

Application difficulties are likely to reveal problems with certain aspects of the problem-solving process (see also Braswell & Bloomquist, 1991). Commonly, children require additional help with issues such as improving their problem recognition skills and being able to see past obstacles to immediate problem resolution.

Concerning problem recognition, many impulsive children don't seem to be able to recognize, or recognize soon enough, the existence of problematic interactions or circumstances. Often, the problems aren't noticed until the child is deeply embroiled. Thus, the child needs additional guidance in learning to recognize problems at their antecedents—when a problem-solving approach is most helpful. This teaching process involves additional discussion and role-play exercises targeted toward the use of available cues to "read" situations. For example, if a client is confused by a friend's negative reactions to the client's well-intentioned teasing, the therapist can guide the child's consideration of the cues that inform us of when it is not a good time to joke with friends. Alternatively, what cues inform us when a friend is in the mood for a jovial exchange? Many application failures seem to be tied to an inaccurate or belated reading of the problem situation, so time spent on problem recognition skills is beneficial in reducing incidents of "failure."

Another common scenario for the disrupted use of problem-solving skills occurs when other people seem to be obstacles to successful problem solving. For example, a child may feel that she has come up with a good solution for resolving a sibling conflict, but her brother just won't cooperate. Or, a boy's effort to resolve conflict with a peer is thwarted by the actions of another peer. To address these and related concerns, the therapist can frame such situations as opportunities for creative, persistent problem solving. Obstacles require persistence. Sports analogies are helpful to positively frame those situations in which obstacles must be overcome. For instance,

T: You've learned to make a jump shot (e.g., be a problem solver) when you're all alone. Now, you're ready to practice the shot (be a better problem solver) when somebody is in your face.

C: Oh, man *(pause)*.

T: No sweat, there are some moves we can try out.

C: OK.

To continue the basketball analogy, the therapist could ask the child what he thinks Michael Jordan would do if Patrick Ewing were trying to block a shot. Would he sit down on the court and quit playing? Sock him in the face? Probably not, he'd just go for the hoop in another way. If football is the sport, we've asked what a good quarterback does if, when he surveys the other team's defense (reads the problem situation), he realizes the play he called in the huddle is not likely to work? Does he stick with the play, walk out of the game because he's mad at the other team, or be a problem-solver who calls another play (an audible)? The therapist can even point out that in most games, not just basketball and football, if you aren't sure what to do you can call a time out to give yourself time to stop and think. Thus, use of age-appropriate analogies can help communicate that everyone faces obstacles to problem solving, it is "cool" to use problem-solving strategies, and it is okay to get yourself out of a situation if you need time to think.

The central ideas behind relapse training are probably obvious at this point—use lapses as opportunities to teach children to bounce back, to cope with the emotional impact of making mistakes, and to use the information communicated by mistakes to further tailor the intervention to the special needs of each child.

GENERALIZATION? BE RATIONAL!

The former expectation that therapy can overcome the child's full array of difficulties and lead to generalized behavioral change is no longer a rational anticipation (Kendall, 1989). Improvements that are evident during and at the end of treatment are to be commended, but they do not necessarily generalize to other behaviors or contexts. Cognitive training, it has been argued, helps a child acquire skills that are transsituational, and the chances for generalization beyond the treatment situations are greater. While the chances for generalization are greater, we cannot assume that the generalization process is that simple. Rather, generalization itself requires training.

One way to ensure that newly learned behaviors will transfer to a second context is to provide some training in the second context. If you desire self-control in the home, some of the training must include thinking through problems that occur in the home situation. If you desire less impulsive classroom behavior, training tasks must parallel tasks in the classroom. Generalization is less a magical process and more a trainable goal. Specific sessions focusing on how to use forethought and planning in new and different contexts are encouraged. Working together to answer the question, "Would thinking about this problem help us solve it and how would I have to adjust what I've learned to make it apply?" fosters generalization.

Another strategy that fosters skill development and generalized application is to work directly to "build bridges." Do not think of the thinking skills as generic, but view them instead as skills that apply in particular domains. Use the child's current level of understanding as the starting place. That is, guide the child through the training tasks by building on what is already known. If a child has managed behavior in one domain, use features of that domain to assist the child in making the generalization. The "dealer's choice" example illustrates this point. Therapists can provide cues—through language, emotional expressions—to assist the child to recognize the similarity between situations. Therapists can structure situations to highlight similarities across contexts. All of these bridge-building efforts are intended to take the child from a place where he/she can inhibit successfully and see how the skills can be applied in other contexts.

Despite the considerable accomplishments made in the development of treatments for overcoming impulsivity, clients do not automatically show gains that are generalized and maintained. Consider this question: "Does therapy cure impulsivity?" Cure here refers to relief, remedy, or successful restoration of a healthy state. Cure is commonly defined in terms of remedial healing that rids one of an illness or bad habit. Cure is not the same as care, which refers to looking after someone who is cureless. Back to the question: Does therapy cure impulsivity?

It can be argued that treatments—successful treatments—teach skills to clients and that these skills are then used by the clients in their ongoing *management* of their psychopathology. In terms of impulsivity, it is not the case that the child will never again be impulsive—such an expectation is irrational. Rather, there will be incidents of future impulsiveness, but there will also be many occasions when the child will be able to use his/her newly acquired problem-solving *management* skills to engage in forethought and planning. It is in the specific teaching of the use of these skills as management skills that we may be better able to improve our outcomes in terms of generalization and maintenance.

COMPLETING THE PROGRAM: DEALING WITH TERMINATION

To the novice, termination means no more than discontinuing the sessions that have been ongoing since treatment was initiated. Quite the contrary is true. Termination is the first effort to determine whether the child has learned and can apply the skills to problem situations on his/her own. Not all first efforts are successful, and readdressing certain facets of the problem may be necessary. Thus, termination does not mean the end of contact.

There are two activities that are a part of recommended termination. First, the child is given a certificate of achievement for his/her mastery of new challenges. All children have learned something, and a positive tone is cast on their completion of the training. Second, as is often done during the last session, the child completes the "SHOWing off" tape. As mentioned earlier, this activity is designed to permit the child to consolidate his/her thinking and to demonstrate to others how the newly acquired problem-solving steps can be used. It is the child's chance to SHOW off, by SHowing Others hoW. Used also in the treatment of anxiety disorders in youth, showing off has great potential as a method to have the child integrate ideas, come up with a fun (creative) commercial, rap song, poem, or the like, and perform it on tape as an ad. Both receiving a certificate and performing and taping a child-created commercial are concrete methods of involving the child in the process of beginning to identify with the merits of the program.

After the certificate has been awarded and the commercial has been taped, there are still matters of termination that require attention. Follow-ups and booster sessions are a part of the posttermination responsibilities of the therapist. How is the child doing in the new classroom? How has he/she adjusted to the new family member? What happened when the child's mother and father fought? Checking up on the child's activities since the formal sessions ended provides the opportunity to remind the child of the thinking strategies, to encourage the child toward higher levels of control, and to reestablish the direct link between real problems and problem-solving skills.

Booster sessions are recommended in two instances. First, and most obviously, booster sessions are appropriate whenever the child has experienced a difficult situation with an unsuccessful outcome. This type of booster session would involve retracing the problem through its stages and rethinking the various actions along the way. Second, booster sessions can be conceptualized as preventive. If the therapist is aware that a child will be shifted to a new classroom, will be receiving a new family member, or is exposed to parental conflict, booster sessions can be scheduled for these events before they become problematic. In either case, reliable follow-ups and timely booster sessions contribute meaningfully to the quality and quantity of the eventual gains that are achieved.

SPECIFIC PITFALLS TO AVOID

Murphy's Law states that "if anything can go wrong, it will." As any coordinator of people, schedules, or activities is aware, things typically do not go as planned. Child therapy is not immune. Children do not attend "key" sessions, parents counter therapeutic recommendations, peer pressures undo long sought after gains, and therapists recognize helpful strategies only in retrospect. The seasoned clinician is all too aware of the vicissitudes of struggling to orchestrate behavioral change.

Cognitive-behavioral strategies are subject to the potential difficulties of all therapies. In an effort to prevent unnecessary frustrations when implementing the self-control therapy, and in an effort to provide helpful hints, we discuss several pitfalls. These potential pitfalls are specific to the intervention strategy outlined thus far and must be added to the already long list that pertains to all therapies.

Missing the Boat: Being Too Focused on the Tasks

Becoming overly tied to the specific tasks used within each session for teaching and practicing self-instructions is a mistake commonly made by novice researchers and practitioners of self-control training. Although difficult, the therapist must remain cognizant that the emphasis of this intervention is on teaching thinking *strategies* or processes and not on teaching performance of specific tasks. Obviously, task performance is learned in the process of acquiring these thinking strategies, but the task is a means to an end, *not* the end itself. In other words, whether the child becomes a real whiz at math problems, tangram puzzles, or even role plays is not nearly as important as the learning of the processes of self-talk and problem solving.

Written correspondence from practitioners and researchers suggests that some implementations of cognitive-behavioral training are perhaps too focused on an exact replication of our efforts. That is, some have expressed a greater desire to copy the exact tasks and less of an interest in replicating the thinking process. One of the jobs of the practitioner is to employ optimal training tasks while emphasizing the thinking skills and processes that occur while engaging in the tasks.

Even with the training tasks available in the *Stop and Think Workbook*, the therapist must still be carefull to prevent an overemphasis on the tasks. For instance, some of the tasks can have multiple answers—two of four choices could be considered correct. In a task requiring the child to think of a word that has a similar meaning, the target word is "loud." Let us assume that the child selects "thunderous." This is certainly a fancy word, and it may be a proper choice, but the therapist was thinking that the word "noisy" was best. The actual word matters little—the fact that some thought went into the response is crucial. A rigid adherence to the tasks might mistakenly lead the therapist to correct the child. But the response—thinking before answering—was not incorrect.

Being too focused on the tasks might be evident in rigid use of the response-cost contingency. The goal is to practice and improve the thinking process, and a response-cost, if applied following a not-so-perfect answer and yet contingent upon careful thinking, would unwittingly detract from the desired goals. Therefore, it is always desirable to ask the child the reasons for his/her choice. If the child did think about the task and produced a reasonable answer, flexible training would provide social reward for careful thinking and point to the other possible answer. A response-cost would not be enacted. The task, and the specific task demands and answers, is again less important than the thinking process. Being eyewitness to thinking deserves, if not requires, encouragement, and the task itself can be sidelined for this higher goal.

The therapist should make explicit statements that draw the child's attention to the transsituational or, in this case, transtask, nature of the self-instructional problem-solving steps. How readily the child actually grasps this notion will be highly dependent on his/her age and cognitive level, but it is still important for the therapist to build bridges and, in essence, "preach" generalization of the thinking processes or strategies.

Didactic "Do's" and "Don'ts": Directed Discovery, Not Dictatorial Demands

Avoid the mechanical or rote use of self-instructions by either the therapist or the child. In learning how to slow down and not answer automatically, the repetitive nature of the self-instructions may render the self-instructions themselves overly automatic. Although it is important that the child has rehearsed the self-statements in order to use them consistently, at the same time, different task situations necessitate variations in the exact wording of the self-instructions. Repeated use of the same catchwords or phrases is important during the child's initial commitment of the steps to memory, but once the child has a basic knowledge of the steps in the problem-solving process, the therapist should think about using variations in his/her verbalizations of the steps.

As discussed earlier, the therapist helps the child translate the self-instructions into his/her own words. The child may nevertheless begin to use the personal phrases in an overly mechanistic fashion. The therapist may then need to coax the child to try out new words and phrases. This may be accomplished by simply asking, "What's another way to say that step?" or "What does the second step mean?" It may also be useful for the therapist to "catch" him/herself being too mechanical in his/her own use of the self-instructions and then model the use of new variations of the old statements. For example, one might state, "Man, I'm starting to sound like a broken record every time I use these steps. I wonder what I could do. . . . I think I'll come up with a new way to say some of these; it will be good to know a lot of different ideas. . . ." In this way the therapist can communicate to the child that not only is it all right to use different words, but, in fact, it is considered a good idea to do so.

We discourage dogmatic or dictatorial demands—the child is never instructed "Say this," "Say these steps," or "Say this to yourself." In contrast, the therapist knows the end goal—thoughtful processing before action—but allows the child to help steer toward the desired goal. The child is shaped into an active, problem-solving mode.

Keeping Therapist Control Issues in Check: Letting the Child Shape the Program

To the extent that it is realistic, it is desirable to let the child experience some control over several aspects of the therapy. A sense of control advances the sense of ownership, which in turn fosters acceptance and use of the problem-solving process.

For example, in addition to not being overly tied to specific tasks, the therapist must guard against being overly attached to his/her own view of what should take place in treatment. Allowing the child to make suggestions about situations in need of problem solving, to adjust the program for personal interests, and to modify or select training tasks can be a simple, yet concrete means of enhancing the child's involvement with the therapeutic process. In a similar vein, modifications in the reward system can be client driven: In one of our child groups a child voiced dissatisfaction with the reward system and eventually cooperated with arranging a solution as part of framing the complaint as a problem to be solved.

To be clear, we are not recommending total child control or anarchy. We view the therapist as continually responsible for ensuring the therapeutic nature of the activities occurring in the treatment context. We do recommend, however, that the therapist be alert to his/her own tendencies, however well intentioned, to "be in control," and not to let these tendencies get in the way of the child's assuming an appropriate degree of responsibility for events and activities within the therapy.

Tension, Upset, and Crisis

Some children may be tense when they come to the therapy session or if and when they encounter difficulties with the tasks. In this case, the therapist might try playing a brief game with the child called "Tense–Relax." The game is intended to help relax the child and is played by demonstrating and asking the child the following:

> How do people look when they're tense and upset? *(Contract all muscles and squeeze up your face)* And how do people look when they're relaxed? *(Let out all the tension suddenly and let your body go limp)*
>
> Let's try this together: Tense *(both you and child tense up)* and relax . . . tense . . . relax . . . tense . . . and relax.

Another game that helps children relax is "Robot–Rag Doll" in which both therapist and child act first like robots (stiff and tense and walking without bending limbs) and then like rag dolls (floppy, relaxed, limp). The therapist might check the rag doll floppiness by lifting the child's arm and letting it drop and showing the child how a floppy arm just flops around when you drop it. These relaxation techniques can be employed when the child is apparently tense, but in most cases these games should be kept brief and used only when necessary. If, however, one is working with a child whose impulsivity appears to be mediated as much by anxiety as by a lack of self-control, relaxation techniques may be made a regular part of the sessions. In connection with these procedures, it could be explained to the child that sometimes when people get worried, tense, or anxious they don't make good choices. They may tend to pick an answer too quickly or jump ahead to another problem before they have solved the one they were working on originally. The therapist's job is to help them learn to make good choices, to teach them some ways to relax, and, therefore, to reduce the amount of tension their bodies are experiencing.

Crises require attention. When working within a structured sequential intervention, the therapist will need to be flexible in order to adjust to the crises that occur. The intervention can maintain its problem-solving focus, but the crisis must be addressed. For example, a 12-year-old girl who was receiving cognitive-behavioral treatment while a patient in a psychiatric day hospital school was sexually abused on the bus to the hospital. When she came to the therapy session, there was only one thing on her mind—the boys who touched her on the bus. The therapist, not a novice with the therapeutic procedures, put aside the assigned session and its tasks but nevertheless maintained a cognitive-behavioral intervention. Following several exchanges, the girl began to look at the incident as a problem to be solved. Several ideas were generated, including the need for an extra adult to ride on the bus, proper punishment for the boys who were involved, sitting in a different place on the bus in the future, and arranging a system for telling the bus driver that his aid is needed. Each potential solution was considered in terms of both long-term effectiveness and present-day satisfaction. A plan was selected and implemented. It was also the case that the therapist made certain that the child did not take responsibility for the boys' mistaken actions. It was not her fault. Nevertheless, she could reduce her risk by sitting in the front of the bus where the driver could hear her.

The specific training materials for the session were not the focus for this therapeutic hour. Rather, the crisis required the therapist's attention and was, appropriately, the problem to be addressed in the treatment. Nevertheless, it was also an opportunity for the therapist to model the use of the problem-solving steps in a real situation.

Rigid Behavioral Contingencies

Flexibility should always be a part of the application of the behavioral aspects of a cognitive-behavioral intervention. In this case, flexibility does not mean inconsistency. Once established, the behavioral contingencies are to be enforced reliably. The particular contingencies utilized with a given child should, however, be tailored or altered to fit that child's needs and should not be rigidly applied in situations in which it is clear that the contingencies are not applicable for that child's behavior. Contingencies are employed to foster and buttress learning, and modifications as needed are appropriate to remain true to this goal.

When we recommend that contingencies be applied consistently, what do we mean by "consistent"? What percentage of the time must a contingency be applied for it to be consistent? When this question has been posed to an audience, some have responded 100%. As you may have guessed, 100% is not correct. A contingency that is applied 100% of the time is rigid and inflexible. For a contingency to be considered consistent, its application should occur with 75% to 85% reliability. It is worth noting that behavior that is acquired under a 100% reinforcement contingency will extinguish more rapidly when reinforcement is discontinued than will a behavior that was originally acquired under a partial reinforcement schedule. This basic feature of learning theory complements our present point—apply the reinforcement contingency with consistency (80% of the time), but avoid rigid adherence to the rules. The following three cases are offered as examples to illustrate this point.

In one of our research studies, three of our subjects were so emotionally distressed by the loss of a chip when a response-cost contingency was enacted that they could not function effectively in the session. With these children, the response-cost aspects of their program were maintained, but, in addition, at the beginning of each session the children were given the opportunity to earn bonus chips by answering simple questions that reviewed the steps and the events of the previous sessions. The therapists used only questions that they felt these children could answer, for the goal of this program addition was to provide each child with a clear success experience that would set a positive emotional tone at the beginning of the session and increase the child's sense of control over the gain and loss of chips. In addition, with these children, rather than simply keeping a written record of the total number of chips they had remaining from previous sessions, we brought in the actual number of chips and gleefully counted them out with each child at the beginning of the session.

This program modification was effective in completely relieving the distress of two of the three children, but a third child continued to show some signs of emotional discomfort. In the face of his distress, we came up with the following modification. We arranged it so that his therapist would allot 20 chips to herself, as well as to the child, and when she was performing problems the child was instructed to response-cost her according to the same rules she was using with him. This provided the therapist with a natural opportunity to model appropriate coping with mistakes, response-cost experiences, and loss situations in general. In addition, it increased the game-like quality of the interaction between the therapist and child, which resulted in a decrease in the child's anxiety in the session. Following this alteration, the child was able to participate, accept response-cost enactments, and in the end express enjoyment of the training activities. Letting the child feel the sense of control that accompanies the dispensing of the rewards (e.g., Stop and Think dollars) has added benefits as well: "You're in charge, and you're doing quite well. It seems like you have really learned how to be a problem solver."

A final case illustrates the potential importance of the backup reinforcers that are available on the reward menu. During a treatment-outcome study, one of the fifth-grade girls referred for training was not responding well in the sessions. Despite valiant efforts on the part of her therapist, the girl persisted in being hostile and resistant to the procedures; she did not seem at all motivated by the potential rewards she could receive. The reward menu included a wide variety of items appropriate for use in the school setting, such as pens, pencils, and folders. This array of rewards was determined to be desirable in the previous treatment studies, but it clearly was not having the intended impact on this girl's behavior. In talking with her teacher and listening to comments within the session, we hypothesized that we had failed to recognize that this fifth-grader actually viewed herself more as an adolescent, and she was insulted by our perception of her as a little girl who would be motivated by the chance to earn such "little kid stuff." Our hypothesis was confirmed, for we found that once we altered her reward menu by adding items geared for adolescent females, such as teen magazines, makeup, and various grooming trinkets, she became quite engaged in the training.

To reiterate the major point, be consistent with the application of the contingencies, but maintain a flexible style. Make adjustments for individual client needs, be humane in the process, and try to keep the response-cost enactment as a cue to go more slowly and keep the emotional sense of reward attached to the reward tokens.

Adaptive Functioning Requires Flexible Thinking

Whalen and Henker (1987) have observed that cognitive-behavioral therapies would probably fare better in outcome studies if these training efforts devoted more time to helping children pinpoint exactly when the use of self-instructional skills was desirable. Most children referred for this type of treatment program have a serious need to improve their capacity to be reflective, but it must be acknowledged that being reflective in every situation is not the goal or the ideal. The therapist can elicit from the child examples of situations in which being "too reflective" would be a problem. If you are about to be hit by a car, get out of the way as quickly as possible. Helping the child recognize the circumstances that require a more reflective approach versus those that do not will increase the probability of effective use.

Discussion of when to stop and think and when to act quickly can result in two lists of situations. With the lists in hand, the therapist can reframe the child's impulsivity as a positive attribute—in certain circumstances. There is no reason for the child to develop overly negative, generalized views of him/herself as dysfunctionally impulsive. Instead, quickness has a place, but an absence of impulsiveness has an important place as well. Making the differentiation allows the child to view him/herself as skilled in certain contexts yet needing new skills in select other contexts.

Therapy Can Be Fun: Prevent the Aversive Context

When the therapy (any therapy) becomes unnecessarily aversive for the child, the outcomes will be less than optimal. And, once the aversiveness has set in, it will be difficult to rectify. Hence, an ounce of prevention is recommended. For example, check that you are allowing the child to have some fun at the start of the session, as well as saving some time for fun activities at the end of the session. Small games, jokes, or any shared activities with the therapist can be fun for the child if managed properly. Therapy needn't be overly serious—as therapists we can lighten up and have fun. As a guidepost, check that your child client is smiling at the start of a session and leaves with a happy face as well. Not that all sessions and all children have to force a happy face, but it is recommended that the therapist use these and other cues to the child's affect as an indication of the child's emotional reaction to the treatment.

Plan to add some fun to the sessions, and arrange to avoid aversiveness. Handling this concern may require some special attention to scheduling. In a school-based intervention program, the therapist should avoid scheduling sessions during recess or any of the child's highly preferred activities. Achieving this goal may require some careful consultation with the child's classroom teacher, for it would also be undesirable to have the child consistently miss class time spent on content areas that are already particularly difficult for that child. Clearly, some negotiation with both the teacher and the child may be necessary, but the point is to avoid cutting the child off from reinforcing activities.

With clinic-based interventions, scheduling may also be an issue. Demanding that the child consistently miss some favored after-school activity in order to come to the sessions will not enhance the therapist–child relationship.

In order to keep the therapy from becoming aversive, it seems to be important to learn how the child's teachers and parents are labeling the intervention. If the adults in the child's life consider the therapy a waste of time or refer to it as something the child needs because he/she is "sick and dangerous," the child is certainly less likely to develop a positive attitude about the intervention. Suggesting that parents and/or teachers refer to the treatment as a special training program that will help the child learn how to solve problems in new ways and avoid some of the difficulties or hassles he/she has been experiencing is highly desirable.

CONCLUSION

Optimizing treatment success is in large part associated with a careful examination of the features of the child client—the specific cognitive deficiencies, the social contexts that are especially troublesome, and the rewards that are potent. Treatment success is also linked to an effective and fluid therapist who applies the program in an emotionally involving and nonrigid collaborative style. Specific recommendations for optimizing treatment impact have been discussed in this chapter:

- Use therapy relapses as opportunities for meaningful skills development.
- Maintain a focus on the training process rather than the training tasks.
- Use self-statements in a flexible, nonmechanistic manner.

- Give the child an appropriate degree of control over aspects of the therapy.
- Train for generalization across tasks and contexts.
- Use contingencies flexibly to serve the goal of fostering learning.
- Point out when a reflective style is desirable and when it is not.
- Attend to the context of therapy and keep it rewarding for the child.

By following the recommendations regarding what features to optimize and what pitfalls to avoid, the therapist will increase the amount of variance in treatment outcome over which he/she exerts control. As indicated by the nature of the suggestions in this chapter, if treatment is to be successful, cognitive-behavioral training cannot be implemented as a formulaic package. Rather, it requires a sensitive therapist who can process myriad subtle variables, collaborate with the child client, and calibrate the intervention accordingly.

CHAPTER 7

Working with Parents, Teachers, and Groups of Children

A s is true for virtually every intervention, the goal of a cognitive-behavioral treatment is to provide knowledge and skills that can be used in the child's real-world environments, such as with friends, family, and classmates. One of the most important strategies for facilitating this type of outcome is the preparation of the child's parents or teachers to recognize and foster the child's newly developing thinking and problem-solving skills. Another means of fostering real-world gains is for the child to be taught the skills in the presence of other children and have opportunities for reinforced practice with peers.

We have several suggestions regarding both parental/teacher involvement and cognitive-behavioral children's groups, but the limits of a single chapter prevent a full consideration of all the specific skills and strategies necessary for competently implementing these methods. For additional discussion, the reader interested in learning more about working with parents and teachers from a cognitive-behavioral perspective is referred to publications by Braswell (1991), Braswell and Bloomquist (1991), Epstein, Schlesinger, and Dryden (1988), Fauber and Kendall (1992), Hughes and Hall (1989), Kendall, Chansky, et al. (1992), and Robin and Foster (1989). Braswell and Bloomquist (1991) and Urbain (1985) provide detailed information about conducting cognitive-behavioral therapy groups with children.

WORKING WITH PARENTS

Although previous cognitive-behavioral efforts with children have varied in the extent to which they included parental participation, the current trend is clearly toward encouraging a greater role for parents. As discussed by Braswell (1991), parental involvement is important for a number of reasons. In some situations, the parent's own issues, behaviors, or expectations may be the major source of the child's or family's difficulties. For example, parental depression could lead to a lack of setting normal limits with the child, and this could result in greater child behavioral disruption. If the clinician were unaware of the parental depression, it would be difficult to formulate an adequately comprehensive treatment plan.

In other circumstances, a parent may not have caused the child's problems but he/she may be making behavioral choices that exacerbate the original difficulties. For example, a child who is predisposed to have difficulties with fear and anxiety is probably not helped by a well-meaning parent who is inadvertently reinforcing the child's avoidance behaviors or promoting confrontation of the feared object in an inappropriate manner (see also Kendall, Chansky, et al., 1992).

In still other contexts, parental behavior represents the major method of impacting the child's concerns even if the parents' behavior has nothing to do with causing or maintaining the difficulty. In the case of childhood autism, for example, parents are not viewed as the cause of this severe difficulty, but special training for parents in the implementation of behavior-shaping methods in the home is considered an important component of treatment.

While including parents is clearly important, it can also make the goals of the intervention process somewhat confusing. Sameroff (1987) and Fiese and Sameroff (1989) have elaborated a transactional model of family functioning that can be helpful when the clinician is making decisions about how to focus the intervention. According to this model, parental/family functioning impacts a given child's development via a three-part process in which (1) a child emits a particular behavior, (2) the behavior triggers a particular parental interpretation, and (3) the interpretation leads to a particular parental response. In a particular case, intervention may need to target any of these three stages. With some situations, it is clearly the child's behavior that is a problem and, thus, the child's behavior requires remediation. In other circumstances, the child may be emitting developmentally normal behavior but the parent misinterprets this as an indication of possible abnormality, so the parent needs help redefining (reframing) the child's behavior. In some families, the parents may interpret the behavior accurately but respond in a manner that is not helpful, so they would benefit from learning more productive means of addressing and coping with the child's behavior. In some cases the treatment must simultaneously address remediation of the child's behavior, redefinition of the parental interpretation of this behavior, and reeducation of the parents concerning reponse options. Clearly, such an intervention depicts a rational integration of cognitive-behavioral strategies.

Form of Parental Involvement

Once the therapist has determined why it would be helpful to have a particular child's parents involved in treatment, decisions must be made about the form of this involvement. To a large extent, the therapy will unfold in accordance with decisions about the content to be addressed and the therapist's preference for how this content should be delivered.

If the primary mode of treatment involves individual sessions with the child, the therapist can choose to involve the parents by meeting with them separately on several occasions to keep them informed about the goals of the child's therapy and to offer suggestions for how the parents can support these therapeutic goals in the home environment. Depending on the preferences of the child, family, and therapist, the same activities can also be accomplished in the context of episodic family sessions. Meeting with the parents separately has the advantage of allowing them to share more openly concerns related to the child, themselves, or the therapy. Family sessions, on the other hand, offer an opportunity for further observation of parent–child functioning and provide a setting for guided practice of any skills that are relevant for all family members. The specific form of parental involvement may also be influenced by a distinction noted by Kendall, Chansky, et al. (1992). These authors note that in some circumstances the parents are viewed primarily as collaborators with the therapist, who provide data and support for the child's therapy, but in other cases or at other points in therapy, the parents may be co-clients, whose own behaviors or beliefs are in need of direct intervention.

Parent group meetings provide another means of parental involvement. Parent groups are particularly desirable when one is dealing with a child condition that has an established body of information that should be communicated to the parents and when the parents are likely to be in need of peer support. Parent groups can be structured to occur independently of services for children or may be coordinated with concurrently meeting child groups. Conducting simultaneous parent and child groups requires the involvement of three to four therapists, depending on the size and the needs of the group(s). In training-oriented clinics or other settings with many therapists, such a format may be relatively easy to structure. In traditional private practices or small group practices, however, this can be more difficult. In such settings, an alternative to simultaneous child and parent groups would be to hold child group meetings for several weeks and then break for a week and during that time hold a parent group meeting. In this way the value of group training could be maintained with a smaller number of therapists.

We urge therapists to think creatively in determining the form of parental involvement that would be most likely to serve the identified therapeutic goals. In a program that will be discussed in a subsequent section, Braswell and Bloomquist (1991) recommend conducting simultaneous child and parent groups for several weeks and then, at planned intervals, conducting separate family sessions with all participants. In this way the groups can be used as a context for learning new skills and gaining emotional support for change, but the family sessions, which can also include siblings, allow the therapeutic content to be further tailored to meet the needs of each family unit.

Content of Parent Training

Just as the exact format of therapy is, in part, dictated by the content to be addressed, the content of therapy follows logically from the functional difficulties of the child and family. Although there is no one correct content outline that must be followed with the parents of all children experiencing difficulties with impulsivity, we do have recommendations for content areas that are typically important for the families of most impulsive children.

Explaining the Purpose and Establishing Realistic Expectations

At the outset, parents need information about the purpose of their involvement in their child's treatment. We let the parents know that while it is possible to help their children learn new thinking strategies in the child therapy sessions, it's up to the parents to model appropriate thinking strategies (and not to model nonthinking) and to reinforce and encourage the use of these strategies in the home environment. In other words, the therapist explains the concept of generalization to the parents. While discussing generalization, the therapist emphasizes a collaborative approach to improving the child's behavior, with the parents actively involved in a team that includes themselves, the child, the child's therapist, and the child's teacher. As part of this introduction, it is important to help parents establish realistic expectations for treatment and treatment outcome. For example, in the case of children manifesting symptoms of ADHD, we make it clear that the child will not be "cured," but using the methods presented in therapy can be expected to lead the child to more effective coping behavior (Kendall, 1989).

At this early stage in treatment, it is also helpful to emphasize that there is no "magic" in the therapy sessions with the children. The child's therapist will be able to teach a more helpful way to think through common dilemmas, but unless the parent takes responsibility for prompting and reinforcing strategy use at home, it is unlikely that the child will display the skills . . . much like what occurs if one attends a foreign language class but then functions in an environment that never encourages or attempts to use the language.

Describing the Child's Condition and Treatment Options

Understandably, most parents are hungry for current information about the condition their child seems to be manifesting, whether it is ADHD, ODD, learning disabilities, more circumscribed impulsive behavior, or some combination of these difficulties. In addition to information about the condition, parents also need expert advice on other available treatments for their child and how these treatments can be accessed. When conducting a parent group, it is easy to devote one or two sessions to presenting this type of information. In the case of ADHD, for example, it has been our experience that parents have particularly enjoyed small group presentations conducted by expert physicians, who could answer their questions about medication, and school personnel, who could advise them about educational options. When working with an individual family, rather than giving them a lecture, it may be helpful to provide them with reading material and then schedule a session to discuss the material and address any questions they have after completing the readings.

With regard to understanding the current treatment, parents may wonder if the training is behavior modification, play therapy, or psychoanalysis. Some discussion of these other approaches is helpful to distinguish the cognitive-behavioral perspective. It is our experience that parents often enjoy discovering what it means to take a cognitive-behavioral perspective. The trainer might even provide the parents with a formal (but understandable) definition, such as the following: Cognitive-behavioral therapy represents an amalgam of the emphasis of cognitive psychology on the effects of thinking on behavior and the emphasis of behavioral psychology on the beneficial effects of performance-based training.

Or, to use less academic language, parents can be told that practice is essential to learning and that their child needs to practice thinking before acting. Other definitions of the cognitive-behavioral perspective appear in graduate texts (e.g., Kendall & Hollon, 1979), journal articles (e.g., Mahoney, 1977b), and undergraduate texts (e.g., Coleman, Butcher, & Carson, 1980). Any definition requires some explication and discussion, but it is important to convey to the parents the joint emphasis on thought (cognition) and action (behavior).

The therapist can point out that one feature distinguishing cognitive-behavioral approaches with children from other types of child interventions is the therapeutic emphasis on *thinking processes*. This focus on adaptive thinking processes is in contrast to the behaviorists' emphasis on teaching specific skills or discrete behaviors. It might also be noted that in stressing the need to modify thinking processes, cognitive-behavioral child therapists teach *strategies* that are designed to be aids to adjustment across a variety of settings. To allay any parental fears that the child's therapist isn't really concerned with behavioral change, the trainer might add that, of course, changes in specific behaviors are considered desirable end products. Selected behaviors are shaped and rewarded throughout treatment, but an essential characteristic of the cognitive-behavioral model is the assumption that it is the training at the level of the cognitive processes that control behavior that will result in the positive treatment effects and their display in different situations. The child's feelings during this process are also addressed.

Presenting Key Behavioral and Cognitive Skills

Following the presentation of information on the child's condition and various treatment options, the therapist is ready to introduce the parents to some key behavioral and cognitive concepts.

Behavioral Child Management

Given that there are many excellent sources on behavioral child management training (e.g., Barkley, 1987; Forehand & McMahon, 1981; Patterson, Reid, Jones, & Conger, 1975), we shall not detail these possible training contents. We will, however, highlight the observation of Gard and Berry (1986) that most respected behavioral management programs address five basic skill areas. These include (1) helping parents increase the number of positive parent–child interactions, (2) training parents to use specific social or tangible reinforcement procedures to increase specific positive child behaviors, (3) teaching parents to use ignoring to decrease mild negative/oppositional child behaviors, (4) training parents to increase child compliance via the parents' use of more clear and consistent commands, and (5) teaching parents to use consequences to decrease inappropriate and noncompliant child behavior. Parents of impulsive children will benefit from understanding how to implement these basic behavioral strategies. If the group leader does not plan to cover these skills and the parents have not previously participated in such training, the leader could help parents identify sites in the community where they can receive such training before moving on to consider the cognitive constructs described in the next section.

Expectances and Attributions

Discussing parental expectancies and attributions can be a useful beginning point for introducing cognitive concepts to parents. In presenting these notions, it can be helpful to first ask the parents to describe situations in which they feel their child expects to fail. The leader can urge the parents to describe the frustrations they feel about the child's "negative attitude" and use these examples to demonstrate the powerful role of expectations in shaping both our feelings and our behavior. Then the leader can shift the discussion to an examination of the expectations that parents have for themselves in terms of their ability to handle the unfolding challenges of parenting a child with special needs. Do they also expect to fail? How might this expectation be affecting their feelings and current behavior toward their child? The goal of such a discussion is to guide the group toward a consideration of the value of adaptive, yet realistic expectations for themselves and their children—not expecting perfection yet not preordaining their failure.

Attributions are clearly related to the concept of expectancies. The therapist can explain that attributions are explanations we create to understand why events happen as they do. While attributions are similar to expectancies, attributions *follow* a behavioral event and are attempts to explain its cause, whereas expectancies *precede* a behavioral event (see Kendall & Braswell, 1982a). In a paper on the application of cognitive-behavioral strategies in the treatment of marital discord, Baucom (1981) discussed how the consideration of attributions and their various dimensions may have relevance for marital therapy. In a similar vein, we believe the discussion of attributions and their dimensions can play a role in child-management (parent) training.

One dimension of attributions described by Abramson, Seligman, and Teasdale (1978) is the tendency to attribute problems or events to internal (within the person) factors versus external (outside the person) factors. To provide an example, parents may attribute their child's problematic behavior to factors outside the child (e.g., a poorly structured environment), or factors inside the child (e.g., neurological impairment). In explaining this notion, the therapist may want to emphasize that it is unlikely that one or the other factor is entirely "right"; rather, as Baucom (1981) noted, the point is to highlight the multiple causation of problems. Parents can also be encouraged to discuss this notion with regard to their parenting abilities. Their unsuccessful parenting efforts could be the result of their own lack of skill (internal factor) or the severity of their child's problem (external factor), and it is most likely to be the result of some combination of these factors.

Another relevant dimension of attributions concerns their global versus specific nature. Global attributions are those that are very general and could apply across a range of different situations, while specific attributions affect only a limited number of situations. For example, one parent might explain a child's poor test performance by making the global attribution that he/she is just too impulsive to perform well on schoolwork. Another parent looking at the same situation might offer a more specific explanation, such as noting that his/her child does poorly on multiple-choice questions because he/she seems to have difficulty pausing to read all the choices before responding. The therapist can point out to the parents that global attributions, although they may occasionally be true, are, for several reasons, likely to be less productive explanatory concepts than specific attributions. Global attributions are typically stated in vague and unclear terms, whereas specific attributions are stated in clear behavioral terms. Also, global attributions can have a derogatory quality and may be anger producing in the child, whereas specific attributions are less inflammatory. In addition, global attributions are often stated in terms that make the problem seem unchangeable, while specific attributions almost provide the prescription for change.

Attributions can also be characterized as stable versus unstable. Stable attributions are those that are less likely to be altered, while unstable attributions are those that allow for the possibility of change. To return to the example noted in the previous paragraph, when a parent notes that a child's difficulties seem to be the result of his/her impulsivity, there is often the implication that this is a stable and enduring characteristic. If one, however, reformulates the difficulty as a failure to read all response options before answering on a multiple-choice test, there is an implication that this specific behavior is not necessarily enduring and may be quite responsive to targeted change efforts. The therapist can explain to parents that although, as was the case with global attributions, there may be some truth to the stable nature of certain causes of their child's behavior, it is usually much more productive (not to mention more hopeful) to focus their attention on those more specific aspects of the child's behavior that can legitimately be viewed as unstable or changeable.

After explaining these notions, the therapist can help parents translate their internal, global, and/or stable attributions about their child and/or themselves into more specific behavioral terms. For example, if a parent has bemoaned the fact that he/she is a poor parent because of lack of patience, the leader can help that parent translate that global, internal explanation into a more specific, balanced attribution such as, "It is hard for me to listen patiently to the children when we are in a rush to prepare supper and the TV is playing loudly." Once a more specific attribution has been produced, the leader can help the group note how specific attributions lead us toward positive steps for improving the situation. In the current example, the specific attribution suggests that the parent might be able to listen better if the dinner hour could be postponed, a simpler supper could be prepared, and/or the TV could be turned down.

Self-Statements or Self-Instructions

Self-statements are another cognitive-behavioral concept that merit some discussion with parents. The therapist might explain that internal dialogues, automatic thoughts, and self-statements are all phrases describing those things that people say to themselves. The therapist could also note that, clearly, self-statements are not independent of the constructs previously discussed. Attributions and expectancies are manifested, at least in part, via the things we say to ourselves, but self-statements can be many different things, including statements of strategies and plans. The introduction of the topic of self-statements and the effort to underscore their universality can be accomplished in a lighthearted manner. The group leader might begin by asking, "How many people talk to themselves?" Most audience members raise their hands, but some will not. The group leader then comments, "Those of you who didn't raise your hands are saying to yourselves, 'I don't talk to myself.'" The routine reaction is laughter as participants recognize the paradox.

To further explain this concept to the parents, the trainer might make the following statements:

> To clarify this notion of self-statements or self-instructions, it is important to realize that we all engage in self-talk at various times. One clear example is when you are learning to perform some new type of activity. Perhaps you can remember when you first learned to drive a car. Most of us began by driving while our parents or driving teacher talked to us and told us what to do. Then we began to talk ourselves through even the most basic maneuvers: "Let's see . . . I have to turn the key in the ignition . . . then I push in the clutch with my left foot and pull the stick back into reverse . . . OK, now I'm ready to back up. . . ." Eventually this self-talk went from being overt to being covert. That is, we quit talking out loud and began to think the instructions to ourselves. Finally, the actions involved in driving became so automatic that we didn't need to consciously talk ourselves through them each time. Other common situations in which adults may notice their self-talk include any circumstance in which the person is attempting to implement a new action, such as learning a new dance, attempting to modify one's swing in golf or serve in tennis, beginning to use a new sequence of operations on one's computer, attempting to assemble those toys that claim to be easy to assemble . . . the list is endless. First we may say the steps aloud and use the words to direct our physical behavior. As we practice the new action, eventually we don't have to consciously talk ourselves through each step. If we do not continue to use the new skill, however, we may find that each time we attempt it we must talk to ourselves again, as we try to recall the steps or actions that once were automatic.

The therapist can then describe the nature of the self-instructional training the children are receiving. It is important for parents to understand that the children will practice self-instructing with many different types of tasks, but the real goal isn't task execution but rather helping the children understand how they can use their internal dialogue to exert greater regulatory control over their own behavior.

In discussing self-instructions and self-control, the leader can help parents establish a developmentally appropriate perspective on these capacities. As addressed in our earlier discussion of underlying theory, we don't expect children to have well-developed, self-regulating internal speech before they have achieved a mental age of 6 or 7 years. Younger children clearly use language to help direct their behavior, but it tends to be the language of significant adults or their own overt language rather than internalized, covert self-speech. These younger children can manage a few simple self-instructions if they are well rehearsed and very specific (e.g., If your clothes catch fire, "stop, drop, and roll," or if there's a bad accident, "call 911"), but they don't have more generalized self-instructional capacities. By the mental age of 7 or 8, however, most children do seem to show more generalized self-regulatory capacities and it becomes increasingly apparent which children seem to be lagging in the development of this attribute.

Problem Solving

Problem-solving capacities are closely linked to the notion of self-instructions and basically involve using self-guiding statements in a manner that leads to effective problem solving. Many different problem-solving sequences have been proposed by various authors, but there are a number of commonalities to these proposals, with most systems including some version of the following: (1) problem recognition and definition, (2) solution generation, (3) evaluation of consequences of each solution, (4) selection and implementation of the selected alternative, and (5) evaluation of the effectiveness of the alternative. Depending on the level of sophistication of the parent audience, the group leader can either list and describe these common elements of problem solving or have the group generate its own list of important components of good problem solving. The leader can then explain how children are learning self-instructional methods to engage in better problem solving with academic and social dilemmas. Other issues related to modeling and prompting problem solving in the home are discussed in the next section.

Through educating the parents about the purpose of treatment, the child's condition, and cognitive and behavioral constructs that are central to the child's intervention, the parents will then have the knowledge base necessary to develop more adaptive, realistic expectations for themselves and their child. In addition, they will be able to more fully understand the importance of their efforts to encourage the child's development of adaptive, realistic expectations toward him/herself. Finally, parents will comprehend the critical nature of their efforts to prompt and reinforce the child's skill use in his/her real-world settings.

Parental Efforts to Improve Treatment Effectiveness

There are a number of steps parents can take to increase the probability of treatment effectiveness. It is our contention that all of the specific suggestions can be thought of as fitting under the general theme of "creating an environment that is supportive of self-controlled behavior." By this we do not mean a rigid, overly structured home setting, but rather a setting in which the adults, as well as the children, have time to think about what they are doing. We are not saying that the hectic, time-pressured existence of many families created the child's difficulties with impulsivity, but we are saying that in order for such children to optimize their functioning, the family's pace of life and choice of activities may need to be altered to permit more time for reflective thinking. With this general perspective in place, the family will then be able to take specific steps to maximize the child's positive adjustment, including modeling reflective behavior and appropriate anger and frustration management, prompting and reinforcing the child's self-controlled behavior, and engaging in collaborative problem solving with the child.

Modeling in the Home

You don't have to be a professionally trained psychologist to recognize that children learn by seeing things done. Children with attentional difficulties or learning problems often have an even greater need to watch someone model appropriate task performance. The therapist can explain that just as verbal self-instructional training emphasizes teaching the child *how* to do a task, the best type of modeling a parent can provide also emphasizes *how* a given behavioral goal is to be accomplished. Often it is simply not enough for parents just to tell the child what they want him/her to do. It is necessary for the parents to show the child what they want him/her to do *and* how they want him/her to accomplish it.

To illustrate this point, the trainer might share the example of the mother who had a difficult time getting her son to put his belongings away in the correct places when he arrived home from school. She tried reminding him to put his things away when he walked in, but this didn't seem to help. Then it occurred to her that her son might not have a clear idea or plan for what it meant to put his belongings in their appropriate places, so for the next 2 days she greeted him at the door when he returned home and actually walked him through the actions required to accomplish this task. She showed him how he could first place his shoes by the door and hang his coat in the nearby closet after placing his mittens in the coat pockets. Then he was to set his lunchbox in the appropriate place on the kitchen counter and take his bookbag to his room. She emphasized the advantages of this method by showing him it took only 1 minute to put his belongings away in an orderly fashion right after school, whereas it sometimes took him much longer to put them away after he had already strewn them all over the house.

The therapist can explain to parents that not only do we know that modeling is an effective way to teach children what we want them to learn, but we also know some factors that increase the chance or likelihood that the child will actually perform the behaviors or actions they have seen modeled. First of all, the type of relationship the child has with the person doing the modeling is an influential factor. If the model is someone the child looks up to and feels warmly about, the child is more likely to imitate the model. Thus, all other considerations aside, a child is more likely to imitate a given behavior if it is modeled by a loved and respected parent than if it is modeled by someone who is disliked or not close to the child. The therapist might grant that there are times when it probably seems as though children would purposefully do the opposite of whatever they saw their parents do, but for the most part parents are powerful models for their children, particularly elementary-school-aged children. If the parents are skeptical of this notion, ask them to think for a moment about how many of their bad habits they've seen their child imitate. The trainer can then emphasize that parents can help their children by realizing what extremely important models they are.

As discussed in Chapter 5, children are more likely to copy a model who talks about or describes what it is that he/she is doing. Perhaps this is because it gives the child a chance not only to *see* the right thing to do but also to *hear* the right thing to do. To illustrate this point, the therapist might state something like, "Your child might learn what to do by watching you correctly solve a math problem or watching you correctly set the dinner table, but he/she is likely to learn more if you also describe your actions as you are actually doing them. In a way, you could think of it as sharing your own self-talk with the child." The group leader can help parents identify common household dilemmas that provide opportunities to model thinking aloud, such as talking one's self through the preparation of a new recipe, fixing some broken household item, or trying to determine how the family will accomplish a long list of errands in a short period of time.

Finally, the therapist can reaffirm that research indicates that children are more likely to imitate what is referred to as a *coping* model than they are to imitate a *mastery* model. As noted in Chapter 5, the advantage of the coping model may be that it gives the child more information about *how* to do a given task or *how* to overcome emotional or behavioral problems that interfere with correct task performance. Of course, it would be silly for the parent to constantly "play dumb" so he/she can be a coping model for his/her child. Nevertheless, each day presents natural opportunities for the parent to be a coping model. The therapist might then state, "For example, say your child is having a hard time fitting everything he/she needs to take to school into his/her bookbag. You have a choice: You could be a mastery model and quickly fit everything into the bag as soon as you see how it needs to be arranged, or you could be a coping model and take a more trial-and-error approach in which you tested out different ways of fitting all the objects into the bag." Again, the coping model seems to be more powerful as a learning tool because it gives the child more information about the *process* or "how-to" part of problem solving.

Prompting and Reinforcing the Child's Reflective Behavior

As previously discussed, effective behavioral child management is important in working with children, but of particular relevance to the current topic is the issue of how parents might use behavioral contingencies to enhance the treatment effectiveness of the problem-solving training. Toward this end, the therapist can encourage the parents to provide social recognition—in the form of a smile or words of praise and encouragement—whenever the child is observed to be making an effort at reasoning through some type of problem. The therapist might remind the parent that a child is unlikely to produce sophisticated reasoning as a part of problem formulations, but fledgling efforts at reflective problem solving nevertheless merit reward. Parents should be encouraged to identify situations in which they might be able to "catch" their child being a careful thinker. One class of such opportunities involves any situation in which the child has to pause and consider a number of alternatives. For example, the trainer might say, "The next time you allow your child to select a treat at the grocery store, try to fight against the tendency to tell him/her to hurry and, instead, comment that you can see he/she is thinking slowly and carefully in order to make the best choice." Parents can be encouraged to take notice the next time their child is puzzling over the rules of a new game and make a remark such as, "I can see you're trying to figure out the right way to play. That's great."

In addition to those happy moments when parents are able to "catch" their child being reflective, the therapist can help parents identify circumstances in which it would be desirable for them to prompt the child to use his or her newly developing self-instructional skills. Often children have a relatively easy time learning the specific self-instructional steps but experience difficulty recognizing appropriate real-world opportunities for using this self-guiding speech. Children need parents and teachers to help them recognize such opportunities. Some families use verbal prompts, such as, "This looks like a good time to stop and think," or "Using self-talk right now would be a good idea." Other families and many teachers also like to decide on a nonverbal signal to cue the child to use the verbal self-instructions.

In some situations it will be necessary for the parents to use aversive contingencies, such as punishment or response-cost, with their children. The therapist can help the parents learn to handle such situations in a manner that might ultimately enhance the child's self-control by emphasizing that the usefulness of such contingencies may hinge on (1) the manner in which they are employed and (2) how they are explained to the child (as well as the extent to which they are consistent). Using the example of "grounding," the therapist might point out that a brief period of time out, such as a few minutes away from a play area, will be sufficiently potent to be a deterrent for young children. Using threats such as "I'll ground you for a month" will only undermine the effectiveness of the contingency, since, almost without exception, parents do not follow through on such grandiose threats. One doesn't need a shotgun to swat a mosquito. Besides, grounding the child for a month tends to punish the parent more than the child.

Time out can also be introduced as a time when the child can calm him/herself down and rethink the problem situation. The therapist might ask the parents which of the following methods of enacting a time out is most likely to foster better problem solving in the child.

> A. "Jim, I've told you 100 times that you shouldn't hit your little brother. You stupid kid. Why can't you act right? Sit by the door and stay there until I say to come out."
> B. "Jim, you are hitting your little brother and that is against the rules in our house. I think you need some time to calm yourself down and get back in control of your own behavior. Sit by the door and stay there until you have gotten yourself under control."

In both examples, the unacceptable behavior is labeled; however, example A also contains insults that may only serve to further hurt and anger Jim. Example B contains no insults and presents the time out not only as a negative consequence for a negative behavior (hitting) but also as an opportunity for the child to "pull himself together" and reflect more on his behavior in order to do a better job. The use of such examples is almost sure to spark further discussion.

One astute client pointed out that taking time out or time to think became a more successful strategy for her child when the parent began to use it with herself. When her interactions with her child would begin to escalate in to a yelling contest, she would stop herself and say aloud, "Stop and think. We aren't able to solve our problems this way. I'm going to go to another room and calm down a bit and I would like you to do the same. Let's meet back here in 5 or 10 minutes and talk some more." By responding in this manner, the mother was able to model more adaptive methods of coping with strong emotions while helping her child take time to reflect on his own behavior.

Engaging in Collaborative Problem Solving

Perhaps the most powerful way parents can assure transfer of skills to the home environment is to go beyond prompting the child's skill use and to actively engage in the problem-solving process with the child. Early in treatment, it can be helpful for parents to collaborate with their child to solve neutral or enjoyable "dilemmas," such as deciding what game to play together, where to go out to eat, what video to rent, or what to serve for a family meal. This provides an opportunity to practice problem solving together without the added emotions that accompany a "real" problem. If these initial attempts are successful, the family can move on to addressing concerns that generate more emotion. To aid this process, some families post the problem-solving steps on a poster on the refrigerator door or some other centrally located spot in the home. If the child refuses to participate in the process, we urge parents to nonetheless continue their problem-solving efforts and involve siblings who are willing to participate. It is still preferable that this problem-solving effort be held within earshot of the refusing child, for we have observed that many children who were initially resistant change their stance very quickly if it appears that a sibling will then have a greater say in a family decision. Clearly, there are family problems, such as issues related to the parents' marriage, that should not involve the children's participation; however, if it happens that the children are already witnessing a dispute in progress, it could be very powerful modeling if the parents attempt to use self-instructions and problem-solving methods to cope with their immediate difficulty.

Summary

We propose that providing parents with new conceptual tools and suggestions on how to think through their own home behavior will foster improvement in their child's problem solving. Of equal importance is the parents' willingness to model reflective behavior, prompt and reinforce the child's use of such behavior, and engage in problem-solving efforts with the child. Facilitating the child's behavioral improvement in the home environment demands parent involvement and support.

WORKING WITH TEACHERS

All the concepts and procedures discussed in the parent education program are certainly appropriate for presentation to the teachers of non-self-controlled children who are in cognitive-behavioral treatment, and cognitive-behavioral teaching/management methods have demonstrated a high degree of acceptance by classroom teachers (Harris, Preller, & Graham, 1990). Given that many children are referred for treatment as a result of difficulties in the school environment, it is usually imperative for the therapist to include some mechanism for school involvement in the child's treatment plan.

In addition to the ideas mentioned in the section on working with parents, there are a number of methods of achieving school involvement. For many clinicians, it is most practical to act as a consultant to the classroom teachers of their child clients. Meyers and Yelich (1989) have discussed the excellent fit between cognitive-behavioral forms of intervention and the requirements of being an effective consultant in an educational setting. For example, as we discussed in the first chapter, the cognitive-behavioral therapist typically establishes a collaborative working relationship with the client and his/her family and just such a collaborative approach is considered important in successful consultation. In addition, effective consultation often involves encouraging the development of more adaptive beliefs and attitudes as well as behavior and, obviously, the focus on both beliefs and behavior is central to all cognitive-behavioral efforts. At a more practical level, serving as a consultant usually involves at least one face-to-face meeting with school staff to share the goals the child is working toward in therapy and determine what skills it would be most realistic to encourage in the school environment. Follow-up telephone calls are helpful in coordinating efforts once an initial plan has been established. The remainder of this section focuses on the ways in which the clinician can serve as a consultant to the educational staff working with a particular client. In other circumstances, however, the clinician might be called on to train school psychologists, social workers, or teachers to become the direct service providers of cognitive-behavioral training for children. Readers interested in such school-based cognitive-behavioral programming are referred to Braswell and Bloomquist (1991) and Hughes and Hall (1989) for descriptions of various intervention programs.

Key Content and Methods

As with parents, it is essential that the teacher be informed of the purpose of the intervention with the child. While the therapist will be helping the child learn new skills, the use of these skills in the home and school settings requires a team approach, with the parents, teacher, and therapist all important team members. After sharing this, the therapist reassures the teacher that he/she is not expected to actually become a therapist in the classroom, but the teacher's prompting and reinforcing of the child's newly developing skills is extremely helpful and highly valued.

Valuing of Self-Talk

Though perhaps obvious, we neverthless note that it is very helpful for the teacher to accept and perhaps even encourage the child's quiet self-talk if the child appears to be using such verbalizations as a means of guiding and directing his/her own behavior in an appropriate manner. The teacher can emphasize the value of self-guiding speech with the entire class by having them identify times when they have observed their parents or others engaging in such behavior. The teacher can note that the way we talk to ourselves can make it easier or more difficult to get the work done. If we talk ourselves through the task and use encouraging language, it will be easier to complete the task, but if we are talking about other things or are putting ourselves down, it will probably be harder. The teacher can then ask the class which example of self-talk would be the most helpful . . . saying something like, "This homework is dumb. I'll never get it right!" or something like, "I need to go slowly and just look at one problem at a time. I can ask for help if I need it." Having the children then give examples of helpful and hindering self-talk allows the teacher to hear the children's own language as they self-direct, and it also provides an opportunity to assess the extent to which they grasp the concept.

Applications with Academic Content

To make self-talk seem particularly real, the teacher might label the attack strategies he/she presents for solving math problems, checking writing assignments, or improving reading comprehension as specific examples of self-instructions that we can use to help ourselves solve particular types of problems. When the teacher is willing to assume a slightly more active role, he/she can help the child implement strategies that result in a better work focus. For example, Parsons (1972) found that if children were required to both name the operation required for a specific math problem (plus vs. minus) and circle the sign of each problem as they began to solve it, their performance on addition and subtraction problems was significantly improved. In our terminology, the tasks of naming the operation and circling the sign made the children truly answer the question, "What am I supposed to do?"

In a similar vein, the teacher might be able to help an individual child develop a short checklist that he/she can use to improve the quality of his/her work in a given type of assignment. For example, questions on a writing assignment checklist might include, "Did I begin each sentence with a capital letter?" "Did I put a punctuation mark at the end of each sentence?" "Did I indent at the beginning of each new paragraph?" As the child's assignments show that he/she has mastered the initial problem areas, new and more sophisticated questions are included on the checklist (e.g., "Does each sentence have a subject and a verb?" "Did I start a new paragraph whenever I began a new topic or idea?"). Ideally, the teacher and student can work together to develop the checklist, with the teacher first asking the child what he/she thinks should be on the checklist. Similar self-questioning approaches can also be helpful for improving reading comprehension. For more examples of specific academic applications, the reader is referred to Ryan, Weed, and Short (1986) and Wong, Harris, and Graham (1991).

Applications with Behavioral Issues

The consultant can help teachers select a few key behavioral issues to address with the child via the problem-solving approach. For example, a particular child may need to work on stopping and thinking before interrupting others or being able to use self-talk to better modulate his/her expression of anger in the classroom. We recommend targeting only one or two behavioral concerns at a time so that neither the teacher nor the child becomes overwhelmed. Additional behavioral targets can always be added once initial goals have been achieved.

The teacher, consultant, and child can then decide (1) on a method for the teacher to prompt the child to use self-instructions (e.g., via a verbal or nonverbal cue) and (2) how the child will be reinforced for successful strategy use. Concerning reinforcement, it is up to the teacher to choose to reward the child's positive strategy use in the context of the regular classroom contingency system or via incentives provided by a home-school reinforcement plan. With the latter system, the teacher sends home a note reporting on the child's degree of success in using problem solving in the classroom on a daily or weekly basis (depending on the needs of the child), and the parents provide a reward for the achievement of prearranged goals.

Behavioral issues involving the entire class, such as frequent fighting over who will be first in line, excessive use of putdowns or name calling (busting or toasting), or difficulty putting up certain commonly used materials in the correct way, can be addressed through problem solving with the entire class. Interested readers are referred to the manual for *Teaching Problem Solving to Students* (Kendall & Bartel, 1990). A teacher can guide the class through each step of the problem-solving process to come up with a new strategy for addressing the particular dilemma. If realistic for the particular case, the child who has received individual training could serve as the "problem-solving leader" for the class. Such classwide demonstrations provide powerful modeling experiences and serve to further legitimize the use of problem-solving self-talk.

Other Relevant Content

If the classroom curriculum includes materials related to social problem solving, such as emotional development programs like Toward Affective Development (TAD) or Developing Understanding of Self and Others (DUSO) (both of which are published by the American Guidance Service, Circle Pines, MN) the teacher could be urged to be explicit about the relationship between these materials and what the child is learning in his/her individual sessions. In such a situation the teacher might point out that learning to recognize feelings is an important part of interacting with others. Being able to identify and label feelings accurately also helps us to identify the emotional consequences that our behavior has, for ourselves as well as for others.

In a similar vein, programming addressing specific interpersonal skills is highly appropriate for many children being treated for difficulties with impulsivity. Such programs often train specific skills such as maintaining appropriate eye contact, expressing feelings appropriately, initiating interactions with others in appropriate ways, and using ignoring appropriately. For more information about various types of social skills programming, the reader is referred to Dodge (1989) and Hops and Greenwood (1988).

Programming designed to prevent cigarette smoking and alcohol and drug abuse may also include elements of problem-solving training that are highly consistent with the methods discussed in this volume. For example, see the work of Weissberg and colleagues (Weissberg, Caplan, & Bennetto, 1988; Caplan et al., 1992) and Elias and associates (Elias, Rothbaum, & Gara, 1986; Clabby & Elias, 1986). The Life Skills Training Program (Botvin, 1983; Botvin, Baker, Dusenberry, Tortu, & Botvin, 1990) was designed to help young adolescents cope with the social influences to smoke, drink, or use drugs by teaching them cognitive-behavioral skills for asserting one's self, managing anxiety, building self-esteem, and resisting advertising pressures. Thus, curricula targeting emotional development, social skills, and drug education can also play a supportive role in improving the child's problem-solving capacities.

Addressing Resistance

As important as it is to have a clear sense of the key content to communicate to school staff, it is equally important to acknowledge and address any indications of resistance or reluctance to implement procedures on the part of school personnel. In our work with impulsive children, we have found several factors to be important in accomplishing this goal.

Typically, the child who is the target of the current efforts has a reputation in the school environment and the school staff may have already expended considerable energy in efforts to help this child. It is extremely important that the consultant be aware of these past efforts and attempt to build his/her current intervention plan based on the success, or lack thereof, of past attempts. As part of this process, it may be crucial to address any feelings of hopelessness or helplessness experienced by the staff in relation to this child and assist the staff to engage in realistic goal setting for themselves as well as the child.

As with parents, helping teachers prioritize behavioral targets to be addressed in the school environment is very worthwhile. The consultant can help the school staff establish a sequential approach to tackling the child's various concerns, so that neither the teacher nor the child becomes overwhelmed with the tasks to be accomplished. In some past school meetings, we have been dismayed when presented with multipage lists of behavioral goals for a particular child and voice concern that to attempt intervention on so many fronts at the same time invites feelings of failure for the staff and the child.

In addition to being aware of past efforts and establishing realistic expectations, the consultant can also point out what the parents or family has been able to achieve or has committed to work on as part of the intervention process. Often, when school staff are aware that the parents are exerting considerable effort to own and work on issues in their domain, school personnel feel more motivated to do their part. Sensitive family information should not be revealed, but with the family's permission, a general sense of the family goals can be shared. Such communication fosters a greater sense of teamwork and shared responsibility and makes it clear that the school staff are not expected to solve problems over which they have little control.

Finally, we find it extremely potent to have the child participate in at least part of the school meeting and to be expected to actively contribute to efforts to problem-solve about specific school dilemmas. This form of participation allows the child to show his teachers the extent to which he/she is capable of talking through difficulties when using a structured format. We speculate that such a display of the child's newly developing skills is probably much more powerful than any explanation provided by the consultant in terms of motivating the teacher to prompt and reinforce the child's use of such skills back in the regular classroom.

WORKING WITH CHILDREN IN GROUPS

We believe that many of the cognitive-behavioral procedures described in this book can be effectively applied in a group setting. The ideal treatment plan for any given child certainly depends on the nature of that child's strengths and deficits, but for many of the non-self-controlled children we have observed, an optimal plan might include a series of individual sessions *followed by* participation in a time-limited group that incorporates cognitive-behavioral principles and procedures. The one-to-one work is needed to allow the child to establish some controls and introduces him/her to the notions of self-instructions and problem solving; the group format provides supervised practice of social problem solving in a setting with peers. Given that the eventual goal is for the children to be able to use social problem solving with peers in naturalistic settings, providing practice in a peer-group context can, arguably, increase the probability of skills transfer to real-world peer interactions. In addition, the group provides an opportunity to practice problem-solving skills with dilemmas arising in a group rather than having to rely on staged or role-played interpersonal dilemmas. In the original edition of this volume, we could offer few examples of cognitive-behavioral group work with acting-out, impulsive children, but there are now many more examples of such work. We shall describe three different programs that include a child group component.

Braswell and Bloomquist (1991) developed and implemented a comprehensive child, family, and school program for working with ADHD children, with child group sessions being one of the key program components. The content of this group is derived from the individual methods described in Chapter 5 of this volume and the group approach described by Urbain (1982). Children are initially introduced to a five-step problem-solving process. In addition, coping with frustration and anger are systematically addressed via modified stress inoculation training (see Meichenbaum, 1985). Using similar methods, children are also trained to recognize and adaptively cope with feelings of boredom. While a structured sequence of lessons is presented to enhance childrens' better understanding of the components of problem solving and coping with uncomfortable feelings, group process is emphasized via "on-line" problem solving about dilemmas *arising in the context of group.* These "group problems" may involve interpersonal conflicts between group members (e.g., two children who attempt to get each other's attention in inappropriate ways), child concerns about the group activities or structure (e.g., group members being upset with some element of the group contingency system), or leader concerns (e.g., not having enough materials or chairs).

In addition to the focus on group content and process, the Braswell and Bloomquist (1991) program involves an elaborated contingency system. The children help designate the desirable group behaviors for which they can earn points and the undesirable behaviors for which they can lose points. The leader reserves the option to provide bonus points for a display of good problem solving by specific members or by the entire group. The group member earning the most points for a particular session is awarded the title of "Kid for the Day" and wins the right to select the free-play activity for the final 10 minutes of group. Extremely disruptive behaviors (harsh putdowns, pushing, hitting, etc.) are addressed via a strike system—if three strikes occur during group, the child must leave the group for a brief period. When this group is conducted in a clinical setting, the parents are meeting simultaneously, so if a child receives three strikes he must meet with his parent and problem-solve about how he can display more appropriate behavior in group. When groups are conducted in school settings, the child receiving three strikes must problem-solve with the principal or some other designated staff person about how he can better manage himself in group.

In their work with ADHD children, Hinshaw and colleagues (Hinshaw & Erhardt, 1991; Hinshaw, Henker, & Whalen, 1984a; Hinshaw, Henker, & Whalen, 1984b) have developed cognitive-behavioral group training sessions that deemphasize self-instructional training and focus more on training accurate self-monitoring/self-evaluation of behavior and anger-management skills. As described by Hinshaw and Erhardt (1991), the self-evaluation training is accomplished via training procedures such the "match game" in which a behavioral goal, such as paying attention, is specified, defined, and modeled. Children are told to think about whether they are paying attention while engaging in the group activities. At a specified point, the children are asked to rate how well they achieved the goal, and they are told to try to have their self-ratings match the rating they think they will be given by the group leader(s). When asked, each child announces his/her self-rating to the group and the leader states his/her rating of that child, being careful to give a very specific explanation of why that rating was assigned. Initially, children can earn bonus points in the group contingency system for accuracy of self-rating, even if they did not do well on the behavioral goal (e.g., they correctly rate themselves as not paying attention). In time, however, the criteria can be tightened to allow bonus points for accurate self-rating and at least marginally appropriate levels of the targeted behavior. The leaders also vary the behavior being targeted for self-evaluation. The anger-management procedures emphasize helping the children to identify their internal anger cues and to learn to monitor the development of their angry feelings. These cues are framed as signals that let the child know that he/she needs to enact some type of anger-coping strategy. Children are encouraged to select a particular coping method, whether it's a certain form of self-talk or an action such as leaving the anger-inducing situation, and then to actively rehearse the use of this strategy in anger simulation role plays.

Lochman and colleagues (Lochman, Burch, Curry, & Lampron, 1984; Lochman & Curry, 1986; Lochman, Lampron, Gemmer, Harris, & Wyckoff, 1989) have developed a cognitive-behavioral group training program for aggressive elementary-school-aged boys. Self-management/-monitoring skills are trained via identification of physiological and affective cues of anger arousal. The children are also taught how different types of self-talk can either enhance or reduce arousal. In addition, in light of numerous observations that aggressive children have difficulty taking the perspective of their victim, this group program emphasizes training the children to more accurately interpret the thoughts and intentions of others as well as to better understand the feelings of others. Social problem solving is also trained, with early problem identification being stressed. The Lochman program includes personal goal setting by the children with feedback on the accomplishment of goals provided by classroom teachers. As was the case with the two previously described programs, ongoing group behavioral contingencies are also an important component of the group.

CONCLUSION

Relative to the time of the publication of the first edition of this book, more researchers and clinicians are calling for the active inclusion of parents, teachers, and peers in the treatment of impulsive, acting-out children. As this chapter indicates, there are emerging ideas about training format and content for use with parents and teachers and the beginning of a curriculum for guiding group training efforts. But, although there are many promising ideas, much more development and evaluation are needed. Nevertheless, there is a consensus that parents, teachers, and peers must be included in the training process if one hopes to maximize the opportunities for the transfer of therapy-trained skills to other settings, the generalization of appropriate responses to other relevant contexts, and the maintenance of skills use over time.

References

Abikoff, H. (1979). Cognitive training interventions in children: Review of a new approach. *Journal of Learning Disabilities, 12,* 123–135.

Abikoff, H., Ganales, D., Reiter, G., Blum, C., Foley, C., & Klein, R. G. (1988). Cognitive training in academically deficient ADDH boys receiving stimulant medication. *Journal of Abnormal Child Psychology, 16,* 411–432.

Abikoff, H., & Gittelman, R. (1985). Hyperactive children treated with stimulants: Is cognitive training a useful adjunct? *Archives of General Psychiatry, 42,* 953–965.

Abikoff, H., Gittelman, R., & Klein, D. F. (1980). Classroom observation code for hyperactive children: A replication of validity. *Journal of Consulting and Clinical Psychology, 48,* 555–565.

Abikoff, H., Gittelman-Klein, R., & Klein, D. (1977). Validation of a classroom observation code for hyperactive children. *Journal of Consulting and Clinical Psychology, 45,* 772–783.

Abikoff, H., & Klein, R. G. (1992). Attention-deficit Hyperactivity and Conduct Disorder: Comorbidity and implications for treatment. *Journal of Consulting and Clinical Psychology, 60,* 881–892.

Abramson, L. Y., Seligman, M. E. P., & Teasdale, J. D. (1978). Learned helplessness in humans: Critique and reformulation. *Journal of Abnormal Psychology, 87,* 49–74.

Achenbach, T. M. (1966). The classification of children's psychiatric symptoms: A factor analytic study. *Psychological Monographs, 80* (Whole No. 615).

Achenbach, T. M., & Edelbrock, C. S. (1978). The classification of child psychopathology: A review and analysis of empirical efforts. *Psychological Bulletin, 85,* 1275–1301.

Achenbach, T. M., & Edelbrock, C. S. (1983). *Manual for the Child Behavior Checklist and revised Child Behavior Profile.* Burlington, VT: University of Vermont.

Achenbach, T., McConaughty, S., & Howell, C. (1987). Child adolescent behavioral and emotional problems: Implications of cross-informant correlations for situational specificity. *Psychological Bulletin, 101,* 213–232.

Ackerman, P. T., & Dykman, R. A. (1990). Prevalence of additional diagnoses in ADD and learning-disabled children. In K. Gadow (Ed.), *Advances in learning and behavioral disabilities: A research annual* (Vol. 6, pp. 1-25). Greenwich, CT: JAI Press.

Alexander, J. F., & Parsons, B. V. (1973). Short-term behavioral intervention with delinquent families. *Journal of Abnormal Psychology, 81,* 219–225.

Allen, G., Chinsky, J., Larcen, S., Lochman, J. E., & Selinger, H. (1976). *Community psychology and the schools: A behaviorally oriented multi-level preventive approach.* Hillsdale, NJ: Erlbaum.

201

American Psychiatric Association. (1987). *Diagnostic and statistical manual of mental disorders* (3rd ed., rev.). Washington, DC: Author.

American Psychiatric Association Task Force on DSM-IV. (1991). *DSM-IV options book: Work in progress.* Washington, DC: American Psychiatric Association.

Asarnow, J. R., & Callan, J. W. (1985). Boys with peer adjustment problems: Social cognitive processes. *Journal of Consulting and Clinical Psychology, 53*, 80–87.

Atkeson, B. M., & Forehand, R. (1981). Conduct disorders. In E. J. Mash & L. G. Terdal (Eds.), *Behavioral assessment of childhood disorders* (pp. 185–219). New York: Guilford Press.

Atkins, M. S. Pelham, W. & Licht, M. (1989). The differential validity of teacher ratings on inattention/overactivity and aggression. *Journal of Abnormal Child Psychology, 17*, 423–435.

August, G. J. (1987). Production deficiencies in free recall: A comparison of hyperactive, learning-disabled and normal children. *Journal of Abnormal Child Psychology, 15*, 429–440.

Ault, R. L., Mitchell, C., & Hartmann, D. P. (1976). Some methodological problems in reflection impulsivity research. *Child Development, 47*, 227–231.

Baker, H. J., & Leland, B. (1967). *Detroit Tests of Learning Aptitude.* Indianapolis: Bobbs Merrill.

Bakwin, H., & Bakwin, R. M. (1966). *Clinical management of behavior disorders in children.* Philadelphia: Saunders.

Bandura, A. (1969). *Principles of behavior modification.* New York: Holt, Rinehart & Winston.

Bandura, A. (1971). Psychotherapy based upon modeling procedures. In A. Bergin & S. Garfield (Eds.), *Handbook of psychotherapy and behavior change* (pp. 653–708). New York: Wiley.

Bandura, A. (1977). Self-efficacy: Toward a unifying theory of behavioral change. *Psychological Review, 84*, 191–215.

Bandura, A. (1986). *Social foundations of thought and action: A social cognitive theory.* Englewood Cliffs, NJ: Prentice-Hall.

Barkley, R. A. (1977). Predicting the response of hyperkinetic children to stimulant drugs: A review. *Journal of Abnormal Child Psychology, 5*, 351–369.

Barkley, R. A. (1981). Hyperactivity. In E. J. Mash & L. G. Terdal (Eds.), *Behavioral assessment of childhood disorders* (pp. 127–184). New York: Guilford Press.

Barkley, R. A. (1982). Guidelines for defining hyperactivity in children: Attention deficit disorder with hyperactivity. In B. Lahey & A. Kazdin (Eds.), *Advances in child clinical psychology* (Vol. 5, pp. 137–180). New York: Plenum Press.

Barkley, R. A. (1985). The social interactions of hyperactive children: Developmental changes, drug effects, and situational variation. In R. McMahon & R. Peters (Eds.), *Childhood disorders: Behavioral developmental approaches* (pp. 218–243). New York: Brunner/Mazel.

Barkley, R. A. (1987). *Defiant children: A clinician's manual for parent training.* New York: Guilford Press.

Barkley, R. A. (1990). *Attention-Deficit Hyperactivity Disorder: A handbook for diagnosis and treatment.* New York: Guilford Press.

Barkley, R. A., Copeland, A. P., & Sivage, C. (1980). A self-control classroom for hyperactive children. *Journal of Autism and Developmental Disorders, 10,* 75–89.

Barkley, R. A., Fischer, M., Edelbrock, C. S., & Smallish, L. (1990). The adolescent outcome of hyperactive children diagnosed by research criteria. I: An 8-year prospective follow-up study. *Journal of the American Academy of Child and Adolescent Psychiatry, 29,* 546–557.

Barkley, R. A., Fischer, M., Newby, R., & Breen, M. (1988). Development of a multimethod clinical protocol for assessing stimulant drug responses in ADHD children. *Journal of Clinical Child Psychology, 17,* 14–24.

Barkley, R. A., Guevremont, D. C., Anastopoulos, A. D., & Fletcher, K. E. (1992). A comparison of three family therapy programs for treating family conflicts in adolescents with Attention Deficit Hyperactivity Disorder. *Journal of Consulting and Clinical Psychology, 60,* 450–462.

Barkley, R., Karllson, J., Pollard, S., & Murphy, J. (1985). Developmental changes in the mother–child interactions of hyperactive boys: Effects of two dose levels of Ritalin. *Journal of Child Psychology and Psychiatry, 26,* 705–715.

Barling, J. (1980). A multistage multidependent variable assessment of children's self-regulation of academic performance. *Cognitive Behavior Therapy, 2,* 43–54.

Baucom, D. (1981). *A cognitive-behavioral approach to marital therapy.* Paper presented at the meeting of the Association for Advancement of Behavior Therapy, Toronto.

Beck, A. T. (1970). Cognitive therapy: Nature and relation to behavior therapy. *Behavior Therapy, 1,* 184–200.

Beck, A. T. (1976). *Cognitive therapy and the emotional disorders.* New York: International Universities Press.

Beck, A. T., Rush, A. J., Shaw, B. F., & Emery, G. (1979). *Cognitive therapy of depression.* New York: Guilford Press.

Beck, S., Forehand, R., Neeper, R., & Baskin, C. H. (1982). A comparison of two analogue strategies for assessing children's social skills. *Journal of Consulting and Clinical Psychology, 50,* 596–597.

Bem, S. (1967). Verbal self-control: The establishment of effective self-instruction. *Journal of Experimental Psychology, 74,* 485–491.

Bender, L. (1938). *A visual motor gestalt test and its clinical use.* New York: American Psychiatric Association.

Bender, N. (1976). Self-verbalization versus tutor verbalization in modifying impulsivity. *Journal of Educational Psychology, 68,* 347–354.

Bentler, P. M., & McClain, J. (1976). A multitrait-multimethod analysis of reflection impulsivity. *Child Development, 47,* 218–226.

Berk, L. E. (1986). Relationship of elementary school children's private speech to behavioral accompaniment to task, attention, and task performance. *Developmental Psychology, 22,* 671–680.

Berk, L. E., & Potts, M. K. (1991). Development and functional significance of private speech among Attention-Deficit Hyperactivity Disordered and normal boys. *Journal of Abnormal Child Psychology, 19,* 357–377.

Bialer, I. (1961). Conceptualization of success and failure in mentally retarded and normal children. *Journal of Personality, 29,* 303–320.

Biederman, J., Munir, K., & Knee, D. (1987). Conduct and oppositional defiant disorder in clinically referred children with attention-deficit disorder: A controlled family study. *Journal of the American Academy of Child and Adolescent Psychiatry, 26,* 724–732.

Bivens, J. A., & Berk, L. E. (1990). A longitudinal study of the development of elementary school children's private speech. *Merrill-Palmer Quarterly, 36,* 443–463.

Blechman, E., Olson, D., & Hellman, I. (1976a). Stimulus control over family problem-solving behavior: The family contract game. *Behavior Therapy, 7,* 686–692.

Blechman, E., Olson, D., Schornagel, C., Halsdorf, M., & Turner, A. (1976b). The family contract game: Technique and case study. *Journal of Consulting and Clinical Psychology, 44,* 449–455.

Block, J., Block, J., & Harrington, D. (1974). Some misgivings about the Matching Familiar Figures test as a measure of reflection impulsivity. *Developmental Psychology, 10,* 611–632.

Bolstad, O. D., & Johnson, S. M. (1972). Self-regulation in the modification of disruptive classroom behavior. *Journal of Applied Behavior Analysis, 5,* 443–454.

Borcherding, B., Thompson, K., Kruessi, M., Bartko, J., Rapoport, J., & Weingartner, H. (1988). Automatic and effortful processing in attention-deficit hyperactivity disorder. *Journal of Abnormal Child Psychology, 16,* 333–345.

Bornstein, P., & Quevillon, R. (1976). The effects of a self-instructional package with overactive preschool boys. *Journal of Applied Behavioral Analysis, 9,* 179–188.

Botvin, G. J. (1983). *Life skills training: Teacher manual.* New York: Smithfield Press.

Botvin, G. J., Baker, E., Dusenbury, L., Tortu, S., & Botvin, E. M. (1990). Preventing adolescent drug abuse through a multimodal cognitive–behavioral approach: Results of a 3-year study. *Journal of Consulting and Clinical Psychology, 58,* 437–446.

Bower, E. M. (1969). *The early identification of emotionally handicapped children in school* (2nd ed.). Springfield, IL: Thomas.

Bradley, C. (1957). Characteristics and management of children with behavior problems associated with brain damage. *Pediatric Clinics of North America, 4,* 1049–1060.

Braswell, L. (1991). Involving parents in cognitive–behavioral therapy with children and adolescents. In P. C. Kendall (Ed.), *Child and adolescent therapy: Cognitive–behavioral procedures* (pp. 316–351). New York: Guilford Press.

Braswell, L., & Bloomquist, M. L. (1991). *Cognitive–behavioral therapy with ADHD children: Child, family, and school interventions.* New York: Guilford Press.

Braswell, L., Kendall, P. C., Braith, J., Carey, M., & Vye, C. (1985). "Involvement" in cognitive–behavioral therapy with children: Process and its relationship to outcome. *Cognitive Therapy and Research, 9,* 611–630.

Braswell, L., Kendall, P. C., & Koehler, C. (1982, November). *Children's attributions of behavior change: Patterns associated with positive outcome.* Paper presented at the meeting of the Association for Advancement of Behavior Therapy, Los Angeles, CA.

Braswell, L., Koehler, C., & Kendall, P. C. (1985). Attributions and outcomes in child psychotherapy. *Journal of Social and Clinical Psychology, 3,* 458–465.

Brief, A. P. (1980). Peer assessment revisited: A brief comment on Kane and Lawler. *Psychological Bulletin, 88,* 78–79.

Broden, M., Hall, R. V., & Mitts, B. (1979). The effect of self-recording on the classroom behavior of two eighth-grade students. *Journal of Applied Behavior Analysis, 4,* 191–199.

Brody, G. H., & Forehand, R. (1986). Maternal perceptions of child maladjustment as a function of the combined influence of child behavior and maternal depression. *Journal of Consulting and Clinical Psychology, 57,* 237–240.

Brown, A. L. (1975). The development of memory: Knowing, knowing about knowing, and knowing how to know. In H. W. Reese (Ed.), *Advances in child development and behavior* (Vol. 10, pp. 103–110). New York: Academic Press.

Brown, A. L. (1987). Metacognition, executive control, self-regulation and other more mysterious mechanisms. In F. E. Weinert & R. H. Kluve (Eds.), *Metacognition, motivation, and understanding* (pp. 65–116). Hillsdale, NJ: Erlbaum.

Brown, R. T., Borden, K. A., Wynne, M. E., Schleser, R., & Clingerman, S. R. (1986). Methylphenidate and cognitive therapy with ADD children: A methodological reconsideration. *Journal of Abnormal Child Psychology, 14,* 481–497.

Brown, R. T., Wynne, M. E., & Medenis, R. (1985). Methylphenidate and cognitive therapy: A comparison of treatment approaches with hyperactive boys. *Journal of Abnormal Child Psychology, 13,* 69–88.

Brownell, K. D., Marlatt, G. A., Lichtenstein, E., & Wilson, G. T. (1986). Understanding and preventing relapse. *American Psychologist, 38,* 1224–1229.

Bugental, D. B., Collins, S., Collins, L., & Chaney, L. A. (1978). Attributional and behavioral changes following two behavior management interventions with hyperactive boys: A follow-up study. *Child Development, 49,* 247–250.

Bugental, D. B., Whalen, C. K., & Henker, B. (1977). Causal attributions of hyperactive children and motivational assumptions of two behavior-change approaches: Evidence for an interactionist position. *Child Development, 48,* 874–884.

Busk, P. L., Ford, R. C., & Schulman, J. L. (1973). Stability of sociometric responses in classrooms. *Journal of Genetic Psychology, 123,* 69–84.

Buss, A. H., & Plomin, R. A. (1975). *Temperament theory of personality development.* New York: Wiley.

Butler, L., & Meichenbaum, D. (1981). The assessment of interpersonal problem-solving skills. In P. C. Kendall & S. D. Hollon (Eds.), *Assessment strategies for cognitive behavioral interventions* (pp. 197–226). New York: Academic Press.

Cairns, E., & Cammock, T. (1978). Development of a more reliable version of the Matching Familiar Figures test. *Developmental Psychology, 5,* 555–560.

Cameron, M. I., & Robinson, V. M. J. (1980). Effects of cognitive training on academic and on-task behavior of hyperactive children. *Journal of Abnormal Child Psychology, 8,* 405–419.

Cameron, R. (1977). *Source of problem solving inefficiency in relation to conceptual tempo*. Paper presented at the biennial meeting of the Society for Research Development in Child Development, New Orleans, LA.

Cammann, R., & Miehlke, A. (1989). Differentiation of motor activity of normally active and hyperactive boys in schools: Some preliminary results. *Journal of Child Psychology and Psychiatry, 30,* 899–906.

Camp, B. W. (1977). Verbal mediation in young aggressive boys. *Journal of Abnormal Psychology, 86,* 145–153.

Camp, B. W., Blom, G., Hebert, F., & van Doorninck, W. (1977). "Think Aloud": A program for developing self-control in young aggressive boys. *Journal of Abnormal Child Psychology, 5,* 157–168.

Campbell, S. B. (1990). *Behavior problems in preschool children: Clinical and developmental issues.* New York: Guilford Press.

Cantwell, D. (1977). Hyperkinetic syndrome. In M. Rutter & L. Hersov (Eds.), *Child psychiatry: Modern approaches.* London: Blackwell.

Caplan, M., Weissberg, R. P., Grober, J., Sivo, P., Grady, K., & Jacoby, C. (1992). Social competence promotion with inner-city and suburban young adolescents: Effects of social adjustment and alcohol use. *Journal of Consulting and Clinical Psychology, 60,* 56–63.

Carlson, C. L., Lahey, B. B., Frame, C., Walker, J., & Hynd, G. (1987). Sociometric status of clinic-referred children with attention deficit disorders with and without hyperactivity. *Journal of Abnormal Child Psychology, 15,* 537–547.

Chandler, M. (1973). Egocentrism and antisocial behavior: The assessment and training of social perspective-taking skills. *Developmental Psychology, 9,* 326–332.

Chase, S. N., & Clement, P. W. (1985). Effects of self-reinforcement and stimulants on academic performance in children with attention deficit disorder. *Journal of Clinical Child Psychology, 14,* 323–333.

Chess, S., Thomas, A., & Birch, H. G. (1968). Behavior problems revisited. In S. Chess & T. Buch (Eds.), *Annual progress in child psychiatry and child development* (pp. 335–344). New York: Brunner/Mazel.

Chiles, A., Miller, M. L., & Cox, G. B. (1980). Depression in an adolescent delinquent population. *Archives of General Psychiatry, 37,* 1179–1184.

Chittenden, G. E. (1942). An experimental study in measuring and modifying assertive behavior in young children. *Monographs of the Society for Research in Child Development, 7* (1, Serial No. 31).

Christophersen, E. R., Barnard, J. D., Ford, D., & Wolf, M. M. (1976). The family training program: Improving parent–child interaction patterns. In E. J. Mash, L. C. Handy, & L. A. Hamerlynck (Eds.), *Behavior modification approaches to parenting* (pp. 35–56). New York: Brunner/Mazel.

Ciminero, A. R., & Drabman, R. S. (1977). Current developments in the behavioral assessment of children. In B. B. Lahey & A. E. Kazdin (Eds.), *Advances in clinical child psychology* (Vol. 1, pp. 47–84). New York: Plenum Press.

Clabby, J. F., & Elias, M. (1986). *Teach your child decision making.* Garden City, NY: Doubleday.

Coats, K. I. (1979). Cognitive self-instructional training approach for reducing disruptive behavior of young children. *Psychological Reports, 44,* 127–134.

Cobb, J. A. (1972). Relationship of discrete classroom behaviors to fourth-grade academic achievement. *Journal of Educational Psychology, 63,* 74–80.

Cobb, J. A. (1973). Effects of academic survival skill training on low-achieving first graders. *Journal of Education Research, 67,* 108–113.

Cobb, J. A., & Hops, H. (1972). *Coding manual for continuous observation of interactions by single subjects in an academic setting* (Report No. 9). Eugene, OR: Center at Oregon for Research in the Behavioral Education of the Handicapped, University of Oregon.

Cohen, R., Meyers, A., Schlesser, R., & Rodick, J. D. (1982). *Generalization of self-instructions: Effects of cognitive level and training procedures.* Unpublished manuscript, Memphis State University.

Coleman, J. C., Butcher, J. N., & Carson, R. C. (1980). *Abnormal psychology and modern life* (6th ed.). Glenview, IL: Scott, Foresman.

Connell, J. P. (1985) A new Multidimensional Measure of Children's Perceptions of Control. *Child Development, 56,* 1018–1041.

Conners, C. K. (1969). A teacher rating scale for use in drug studies with children. *American Journal of Psychiatry, 126,* 884–888.

Conners, C. K. (1970). Symptom patterns in hyperkinetic, neurotic, and normal children. *Child Development, 41,* 667–682.

Conners, C. K. (1973). What parents need to know about stimulant drugs and special education. *Journal of Learning Disabilities, 6,* 13–15.

Conners, C. K. (1980). *Food additives and hyperactive children.* New York: Plenum Press.

Conrad, W., & Insel, J. (1967). Anticipating the response to amphetamine therapy in the treatment of hyperkinetic children. *Pediatrics, 40,* 96–98.

Copeland, A. P. (1983). Children's talking to themselves: Its developmental significance, function, and therapeutic promise. In P. C. Kendall (Ed.), *Advances in cognitive behavioral research and therapy* (Vol. 2, pp. 242–279). New York: Academic Press.

Costello, A. J., Edelbrock, C., Kalas, R., Dulcan, M. & Klaric, S. (1984). *Development and testing of the NIMH Diagnostic Interview Schedule for Children (DISC) in a clinic population: Final report.* Rockville, MD: Center for Epidemiological Studies, NIMH.

Cowen, E. L., Pederson, A., Babigian, H., Izzo, L., & Trost, M. A. (1973). Long-term follow-up of early detected vulnerable children. *Journal of Consulting and Clinical Psychology, 41,* 438–446.

Craighead, W. E. (1982). A brief clinical history of cognitive–behavioral therapy with children. *School Psychology Review, 11,* 5–13.

Crandall, U. C., Katkovsky, W., & Crandall, V. G. (1965). Children's beliefs in their own control of reinforcement in intellectual academic achievement situations. *Child Development, 36,* 91–109.

Cullinan, D., Epstein, M. H., & Silver, L. (1977). Modification of impulsive tempo in learning-disabled pupils. *Journal of Abnormal Child Psychology, 5,* 437–444.

Curry, J. F., & Craighead, W. E., (1990). Attributional style in clinically depressed and conduct-disordered adolescents. *Journal of Consulting and Clinical Psychology, 58,* 109–116.

Dadds, M. R., Schwartz, S., & Sanders, M. R. (1987). Marital discord and treatment outcome in behavioral treatment of child conduct disorders. *Journal of Consulting and Clinical Psychology, 55,* 396–403.

Day, A. M. L., & Peters, R. D. (1989). Assessment of attentional difficulties in underachieving children. *Journal of Educational Research, 82,* 356–361.

Delfini, L. F., Bernal, M. E., & Rosen, P. M. (1976). Comparison of deviant and normal boys in home settings. In E. J. Mash, L. A. Hamerlynck, & L. C. Handy (Eds.), *Behavior modification and families* (pp. 228–248). New York: Brunner/Mazel.

Denhoff, E. (1973). The natural life history of children with minimal brain dysfunction. *Annals of the New York Academy of Science, 205,* 188–205.

Dobson, K. S. (Ed.). (1988). *Handbook of cognitive–behavioral therapies.* New York: Guilford Press.

Dodge, K. A. (1980). Social cognition and children's aggressive behavior. *Child Development, 51,* 162–170.

Dodge, K. A. (1989). Problems in social relationships. In E. J. Mash & R. A. Barkley (Eds.), Treatment of childhood disorders (pp. 222–244). New York: Guilford Press.

Dodge, K. A., & Newman, J. P. (1981). Biased decision-making processes in aggresive boys. *Journal of Abnormal Psychology, 90,* 375–379.

Dodge, K. A., Pettit, G. S., McClaskey, C. L., & Brown, M. M. (1986). Social competence in children. *Monographs of the Society for Research in Child Development, 51,* (2, Serial No. 213).

Douglas, V. I. (1980). Higher mental processes in hyperactive children: Implications for training. In R. M. Knights & D. J. Bakker (Eds.), *Treatment of hyperactive and learning disordered children* (pp. 65–92). Baltimore, MD: University Park.

Douglas, V.I. (1983). Attentional and cognitive problems. In M. Rutter (Ed.), *Developmental neuropsychiatry* (pp. 280–320). New York: Guilford Press.

Douglas, V. I., Parry, P., Marton, P., & Garson, C. (1976). Assessment of a cognitive training program for hyperactive children. *Journal of Abnormal Child Psychology, 4,* 389–410.

Douglas, V. I., & Peters, K. G. (1979). Toward a clearer definition of the attentional deficit of hyperactive children. In G. A. Hale & M. Lewis (Eds.), *Attention and the development of cognitive skills* (pp. 173–248). New York: Plenum Press.

Drabman, R. S., Spitalnik, R., & O'Leary, K. D. (1973). Teaching self-control to disruptive children. *Journal of Abnormal Psychology, 82,* 10–16.

Dubow, E. F., Huesmann, L. R., & Eron, L. D. (1987). Mitigating aggression: Promoting prosocial behavior in aggressive elementary schoolboys. *Behavior Research and Therapy, 24,* 227–230.

Dunn, L. M. (1965). *Expanded manual for the Peabody Picture Vocabulary Test.* Minneapolis, MN: American Guidance Services.

Durrell, D. D. (1955). *Durrell Analysis of Reading Difficulty.* New York: Harcourt, Brace & World.

Dush, D. M., Hirt, M. L., & Schroeder, H. E. (1989). Self-statement modification in the treatment of child behavior disorders: A meta-analysis. *Psychological Bulletin, 106,* 97–106.

D'Zurilla, T. J. (1986). *Problem-solving therapy: A social competence approach to clinical intervention.* New York: Springer.

D'Zurilla, T. J., & Goldfried, M. R. (1971). Problem solving and behavior modification. *Journal of Abnormal Psychology, 78,* 107–126.

D'Zurilla, T. J., & Nezu, A. (1982). Social problem solving in adults. In P. C. Kendall (Ed.), *Advances in cognitive–behavioral research and therapy* (Vol. 1, pp. 202–275). New York: Academic Press.

Edelbrock, C. S. (1985). *Conduct problems in childhood and adolescence: Developmental patterns and progressions.* Unpublished manuscript.

Edelbrock, C. & Costello, A. (1988). Convergence between statistically derived behavior problem syndromes and child psychiatric diagnoses. *Journal of Abnormal Child Psychology, 16,* 219–231.

Edelbrock, C. S., Costello, A., Dulcan, M. J., Conover, N. C., & Kalas, R. (1986). Parent-child agreement of child psychiatric symptoms assessed via structured interview. *Journal of Child Psychology and Psychiatry, 27,* 181–190.

Edelbrock, C., Greenbaum, R., & Conover, N. (1985). Reliability and concurrent relations between the teacher version of the Child Behavior Profile and the Conners Revised Teacher Rating Scale. *Journal of Abnormal Child Psychology, 13,* 295–304.

Egeland, B., Bielke, P., & Kendall, P. C. (1980). Achievement and adjustment correlates of the Matching Familiar Figures test. *Journal of School Psychology, 18,* 361–372.

Egeland, B., & Weinberg, R. A. (1976). The Matching Familiar Figures test: A look at its psychometric credibility. *Child Development, 47,* 483–491.

Elias, M. J., & Branden, L. R. (1988). Primary prevention of behavioral and emotional problems in school-aged populations. *School Psychology Review, 17,* 581–592.

Elias, M. J., Rothbaum, P. A., & Gara, M. (1986) Social–cognitive problem solving in children: Assessing the knowledge and application of skills. *Journal of Applied and Developmental Psychology, 7,* 77–94.

Elkin, A. (1983). Group work with children and youth. In A. Ellis & M. E. Bernard (Eds.), Rational–emotive approaches to the problems of childhood (pp. 485–508). New York: Plenum Press.

Ellis, A. (1962). *Reason and emotion in psychotherapy.* New York: Stuart.

Emery, R. E. (1982). Interparental conflict and the children of discord and divorce. *Psychological Bulletin, 92,* 310–330.

Enright, R. D. (1977). *Social cognitive development: A training model for intermediate school-age children.* St. Paul, MN: Pupil Personnel Division, Minnesota State Department of Education.

Epps, J., Ronan, K.R., & Kendall, P. C. (1990). *Moderator variables in a cognitive–behavioral treatment for conduct-disordered children.* Unpublished manuscript, Temple University, Philadelphia.

Epstein, N. E., Schlesinger, S. E., & Dryden, W. (1988). Concepts and methods of cognitive-behavior family treatment. In N. Epstein, S. Schlesinger, & W. Dryden (Eds.), *Cognitive–behavioral therapy with families* (pp. 5–48). New York: Brunner/Mazel.

Fauber, R., & Kendall, P. C. (1992). Children and families: Integrating the focus of intervention. *Journal of Psychotherapy Integration, 2,* 107–123.

Feindler, E. L. (1991). Cognitive strategies in anger control interventions for children and adolescents. In P. C. Kendall (Ed.), *Child and adolescent therapy: Cognitive–behavioral procedures* (pp. 66–97). New York: Guilford Press.

Feindler, E. L., Ecton, R. B., Kingsley, D., & Dubey, D. (1986). Group anger control training for institutionalized psychiatric male adolescents. *Behavior Therapy, 17,* 109–123.

Feldhusen, J., & Houtz, J. (1975). Problem solving and the concrete–abstract dimension. *Gifted Child Quarterly, 19,* 122–129.

Feldhusen, J., Houtz, J., & Ringenbach, S. (1972). The Purdue Elementary Problem-Solving Inventory. *Psychological Reports, 31,* 891–901.

Fiese, B. H., & Sameroff, A. J. (1989). Family context in pediatric psychology: A transactional perspective. *Journal of Pediatric Psychology, 14,* 293–314.

Finch, A. J. Jr., Kendall, P. C., Deardorff, P. A., Anderson, J., & Sitarz, A. M. (1975a). Reflection impulsivity, persistence behavior, and locus of control in emotionally disturbed children. *Journal of Consulting and Clinical Psychology, 43,* 748.

Firestone, P. (1982). Factors associated with children's adherence to stimulant medication. *American Journal of Orthopsychiatry, 52,* 447–457.

Fischer, M., Barkley, R. A., Edelbrock, C. S., & Smallish, L. (1990). The adolescent outcome of hyperactive children diagnosed by research criteria, II: Academic, attentional and neuropsychological status. *Journal of Consulting and Clinical Psychology, 58,* 580–588.

Fischler, G., & Kendall, P. C. (1988). Social cognitive problem solving and childhood adjustment: Qualitative and topological analyses. *Cognitive Therapy and Research, 12,* 133–154.

Fish, B. (1971). The "one child, one drug" myth of stimulants in hyperkinesis. *Archives of General Psychiatry, 25,* 193–203.

Flavell, J. H. (1976). Metacognitive aspects of problem solving. In L. B. Resnick (Ed.), *The nature of intelligence* (pp. 231–296). Hillsdale, NJ: Erlbaum.

Flavell, J. H. (1977). *Cognitive development.* Englewood Cliffs, NJ: Prentice-Hall.

Forehand, R., King, H. E., Peed, S., & Yoder, P. (1975). Mother–child interactions: Comparison of a noncompliant clinic group and a nonclinic group. *Behaviour Research and Therapy, 13,* 79–84.

Forehand, R. L., & McMahon, R. J. (1981). *Helping the noncompliant child: A clinician's guide to parent training.* New York: Guilford Press.

Foster, S. L. (1979). Family conflict management: Skill training and generalization procedures. *Dissertation Abstracts International, 39,* 5063B–5064B. (University Microfilms No. 79-08, 689)

Foster, S. L., & Robin, A. L. (1989). Parent–adolescent conflict. In E. J. Mash & R. J. Barkley (Eds.), *Treatment of childhood disorders* (pp. 493–528). New York: Guilford Press.

Frick, P. J., Kamphaus, R. W., Lahey, B. B., Loeber, R., Christ, M. A., Hart, E. L., & Tannenbaum, L. E. (1991). Academic underachievement and the Disruptive Behavior Disorders. *Journal of Consulting and Clinical Psychology, 59,* 289–294.

Friedling, C., & O'Leary, S. G. (1979). Effects of self-instructional training on second- and third-grade hyperactive children: A failure to replicate. *Journal of Applied Behavior Analysis, 12,* 211–219.

Gaddis, L. R., & Martin, R. P. (1989). Relationship among measures of impulsivity for preschoolers. *Journal of Psychoeducational Assessment, 7,* 284–295.

Gal'perin, P. Y. (1969). Stages in the development of mental acts. In M. Cole & I. Maltzman (Eds.), *A handbook of contemporary Soviet psychology* (pp. 249–273). New York: Basic Books.

Gard, G. C., & Berry, K. K. (1986). Oppositional children: Training tyrants. *Journal of Clinical Child Psychology, 15,* 148–158.

Giebink, J. W., Stover, D., & Fahl, M. (1968). Teaching adaptive responses to frustration to emotionally disturbed boys. *Journal of Consulting and Clinical Psychology, 32,* 366–368.

Glueck, S., & Glueck, E. T. (1950). *Unraveling juvenile delinquency.* New York: Commonwealth Fund.

Golden, M., Montane, A., & Bridger, W. (1977). Verbal control of delay behavior in two-year-old boys as a function of social class. *Child Development, 48,* 1107–1111.

Goodwin, S., & Mahoney, M. J. (1975). Modification of aggression through modeling: An experimental probe. *Journal of Behavior Therapy and Experimental Psychiatry, 6,* 200–202.

Gordon, D. A., & Arbuthnot, J. (1987). Individual, group and family interventions. In H. C. Quay (Ed.), *Handbook of juvenile delinquency* (pp. 290-324). New York: Wiley.

Gordon, T. (1970). *Parent effectiveness training.* New York: Wyden.

Goyette, C. H., Conners, C. K., & Ulrich, R. F. (1978). Normative data on revised Conners Parent and Teacher Rating Scales. *Journal of Abnormal Child Psychology, 6,* 221–236.

Graham, L. (1986). *The comparative effectiveness of didactic teaching and self-instructional training of a question-answering strategy in enhanced reading comprehension.* Unpublished master's thesis, Simon Fraser University, Burnaby, British Columbia, Canada.

Graham, S., & Harris, K. R. (1989a) A components analysis of cognitive strategy instruction: Effects on learning-disabled students' compositions and self-efficacy. *Journal of Educational Psychology, 81,* 353–361.

Graham, S., & Harris, K. R. (1989b). Improving learning-disabled students' skills at composing essays: Self-instructional strategy training. *Exceptional Children, 56,* 201–214.

Graves, A. W. (1986). Effects of direct instruction and metacomprehension on finding main ideas. *Learning Disability Research, 1,* 90–100.

Griest, D. L., Forehand, R., Rogers, T., Breiner, J., Furey, W., & Williams, C. A. (1982). Effects of parent enhancement therapy on the treatment outcome and generalization of a parent training program. *Behaviour Research and Therapy, 20,* 429–436.

Guevremont, D.C., DuPaul, G. J., & Barkley, R. A. (1990). Diagnosis and assessment of Attention-Deficit Hyperactivity Disorder in children. *Journal of School Psychology, 28,* 51–78.

Guralnick, M. J. (1976). Solving complex perceptual discrimination problems: Techniques for the development of problem-solving strategies. *American Journal of Mental Deficiency, 81,* 18–25.

Gurucharri, C., Phelps, E., & Selman, R. (1984). Development of interpersonal understanding: A longitudinal and comparative study of normal and disturbed youths. *Journal of Consulting and Clinical Psychology, 52,* 26–36.

Harlow, H. F., & Mears, C. (1979). *The human model: Primate perspectives.* New York: Wiley.

Harris, K. R. (1986a). The effects of cognitive–behavior modification on private speech and task performance during problem solving among learning-disabled and normally achieving children. *Journal of Abnormal Child Psychology, 14,* 63–67.

Harris, K. R. (1986b). Self-monitoring of attentional behavior versus self-monitoring of productivity: Effects on on-task behavior and academic response rate among learning-disabled children. *Journal of Applied Behavior Analysis, 19,* 417–423.

Harris, K. R., & Graham., S (1985). Improving learning-disabled students' composition skills: Self-control strategy training. *Learning Disability Quarterly, 8,* 27–36.

Harris, K. R., & Graham, S. (1988). Self-instructional strategy training: Improving writing skills among educationally handicapped students. *Teaching Exceptional Students, 20,* 35–37.

Harris, K. R., Preller, D., M., & Graham, S. (1990). Acceptability of cognitive–behavioral and behavioral interventions among teachers. *Cognitive Therapy and Research, 14,* 573–587.

Harter, S. (1979, October). *A model of intrinsic motivation in children: Individual differences and developmental change.* Invited address presented at the Minnesota Symposium on Child Psychology, Minneapolis.

Harter, S. (1982). The Perceived Competence Scale for Children. *Child Development, 53,* 87–97.

Harter, S. (1985). *The Self-Perception Profile for Children: Revision of the Perceived Competence Scale for Children (Manual).* Denver, CO: University of Denver.

Hartsough, C. S., & Lambert, N. M. (1982). Some environmental and familial correlates and antecedents of hyperactivity. *American Journal of Orthopsychiatry, 52,* 272–287.

Hartsough, C. S., & Lambert, N. M. (1984). Contribution of predispositional factors to the diagnosis of hyperactivity. *American Journal of Orthopsychiatry, 54,* 97–109.

Hartsough, C. S., & Lambert, N. M. (1985). Medical factors in hyperactive and normal children: Prenatal, developmental and health history findings. *American Journal of Orthopsychiatry, 55,* 190–201.

Hartup, W. W. (1983). Peer relations. In P. Mussen (Ed.), *Handbook of child psychology* (4th ed.) (Vol. 4, pp. 361–456). New York: Wiley.

Haynes, S. N. (1978). *Principles of behavioral assessment.* New York: Gardner.

Hechtman, L., Weiss, G., Finkelstein, J., Wener, A., & Benn, R. (1976). Hyperactives as young adults. Preliminary report. *Canadian Medical Association Journal, 115,* 625–630.

Henggeler, S. W., Melton, G. B., & Smith, L. A. (1992). Multisystemic treatment of serious juvenile offenders: An effective alternative to incarceration. *Journal of Consulting and Clinical Psychology, 60,* 953–961.

Herjanic, B., & Reich, W. (1982). Development of a structured psychiatric interview for children: Agreement between child and parent on individual symptoms. *Journal of Abnormal Child Psychology, 10,* 307–324.

Hinshaw, S. P. (1987). On the distinction between attentional deficits/hyperactivity and conduct problems/aggression in child psychopathology. *Psychological Bulletin, 101,* 443–463.

Hinshaw, S. P., & Erhardt, D. (1991). Attention-deficit Hyperactivity Disorder. In P. C. Kendall (Ed.), *Child and adolescent therapy: Cognitive–behavioral procedures* (pp. 98–128). New York: Guilford Press.

Hinshaw, S. P., Henker, B., & Whalen, C. K. (1984a). Cognitive–behavioral and pharmacologic interventions for hyperactive boys: Comparative and combined effects. *Journal of Consulting and Clinical Psychology, 52,* 739–749.

Hinshaw, S. P., Henker, B., & Whalen, C. K. (1984b). Self-control in hyperactive boys in anger-inducing situations: Effects of cognitive–behavioral training and of methylphenidate. *Journal of Abnormal Child Psychology, 12,* 55–77

Hobbs, S. A., Moquin, L. E., Tyroler, M., & Lahey, B. B. (1980). Cognitive-behavior therapy with children: Has clinical utility been demonstrated? *Psychological Bulletin, 87,* 147–165.

Hogan, A. E., Quay, H. C., Vaughn, S., & Shapiro, S. K. (1989). Revised Behavior Problem Checklist: Stability, prevalence, and incidence of behavior problems in kindergarten and first-grade children. *Psychological Assessment: A Journal of Consulting and Clinical Psychology, 1,* 103–111.

Homatidis, S., & Konstantareas, M. M. (1981). Assessment of hyperactivity: Isolating measures of high discriminant validity. *Journal of Consulting and Clinical Psychology, 49,* 533–541.

Hooper, S. R., & Willis, W. G. (1989). *Learning disability subtyping: Neuropsychological foundations, conceptual models, and issues in clinical differentiation.* New York: Springer-Verlag.

Hops, H. & Greenwood, C. R. (1988). Social skills deficits. In E. J. Mash & L. G. Terdal (Eds.), *Behavioral assessment of childhood disorders* (2nd ed.) (pp. 263–314). New York: Guilford Press.

Hoy, E., Weiss, G., Minde, K., & Cohen, N. (1978). The hyperactive child at adolescence: Cognitive, emotional, and social functioning. *Journal of Abnormal Child Psychology, 67,* 311–324.

Huessy, H. R. (1974). Hyperkinetic problems continue to teens. *Clinical Psychiatry News, 2,* 5.

Hughes, J. N., & Hall, R. J. (Eds.). (1989). *Cognitive–behavioral psychology in the schools: A comprehensive handbook.* New York: Guilford Press.

Ingram, R. E. (Ed.). (1986). *Information-processing approaches to clinical psychology.* New York: Academic Press.

Ingram, R. E., & Kendall, P. C. (1986). Cognitive clinical psychology: Implications of an information-processing perspective. In R. E. Ingram (Ed.), *Information-processing approaches to clinical psychology* (pp. 3–21). New York: Academic Press.

Institute of Medicine. (1989). *Research on children and adolescents with mental, behavioral, and devlopmental disorders.* Washington, DC: National Academy Press.

Jacob, R. G., O'Leary, K. D., & Rosenblad, C. (1978). Formal and informal classroom settings: Effects on hyperactivity. *Journal of Abnormal Child Psychology, 6,* 47–60.

Jahoda, M. (1953). The meaning of psychological health. *Social Casework, 34,* 349–354.

Jahoda, M. (1958). *Current concepts of positive mental health.* New York: Basic Books.

Jastak, J. F., Bijou, S. W., & Jastak, S. R. (1965). *Wide Range Achievement Test.* Wilmington, DE: Guidance Associates.

Jensen, J. B., Burke, N., & Garfinkel, B. D. (1988). Depression and symptoms of attentional deficit disorder with hyperactivity. *Journal of the American Academy of Child and Adolescent Psychiatry, 27,* 742–747.

Johnson, S. M., Bolstad, O. D., & Lobitz, G. K. (1976). Generalization and contrast phenomena in behavior modification with children. In E. J. Mash, L. A. Hamerlynck, & L. C. Handy (Eds.), *Behavior modification and families* (pp. 160–188). New York: Brunner/Mazel.

Johnson, S. M., & Lobitz, G. K. (1974). The personal and marital status of parents as related to observed child deviance and parenting behaviors. *Journal of Abnormal Child Psychology, 3,* 193–208.

Johnston, M. B., Whitman, T. L., & Johnson, M. (1980). Teaching addition and subtraction to mentally retarded children: A self-instruction program. *Applied Research in Mental Retardation, 1,* 141–160.

Jones, R. N., Latkowski, M., Kircher, J., & McMahon, W. M. (1988). The Child Behavior Checklist: Normative information for inpatients. *Journal of the American Academy of Child and Adolescent Psychiatry, 27,* 632–635.

Jouriles, E. N., Pfiffner, L. J., & O'Leary, S. G. (1988). Marital conflict, parenting, and toddler conduct problems. *Journal of Abnormal Child Psychology, 16,* 197–206.

Kagan, J. (1965). Reflection-impulsivity and reading ability in primary grade children. *Child Development, 36,* 609–628.

Kagan, J. (1966). Reflection-impulsivity: The generality and dynamics of conceptual tempo. *Journal of Abnormal Psychology, 71,* 17–24.

Kagan, J., & Messer, S. B. (1975). A reply to "Some misgivings about the Matching Familiar Figures test as a measure of impulsivity." *Developmental Psychology, 11,* 244–248.

Kagan, J., Rosman, B. L., Day, D., Albert, J., & Phillips, W. (1964). Information processing in the child: Significance of analytic and reflective attitudes. *Psychological Monographs, 78* (1, Whole No. 578).

Kamann, M. P. (1989). *Inducing adaptive coping self-statements in the learning-disabled through a cognitive behavioral intervention.* Unpublished master's thesis, Simon Fraser University, Burnaby, British Columbia, Canada.

Kane, J. S., & Lawler, E. E. (1978). Methods of peer assessment. *Psychological Bulletin, 85,* 555–586.

Kanfer, F. H. (1970). Self-regulation: Research issues and speculations. In C. Nuringer & J. L. Michael (Eds.), *Behavior modification in clinical psychology* (pp. 178–220). New York: Appleton-Century-Crofts.

Karoly, P. (1981). Self-management problems in children. In E. J. Mash & L. G. Terdal (Eds.), *Behavioral assessment of childhood disorders* (pp. 79–126). New York: Guilford Press.

Kazdin, A. E. (1974). Covert modeling, model similarity, and reduction of avoidance behavior. *Behavior Therapy, 5,* 325–340.

Kazdin, A. E. (1987). Treatment of antisocial behavior in children: Current status and furture directions. *Psychological Bulletin, 102,* 187–203.

Kazdin, A. E., Bass, D., Siegel, T., & Thomas, C. (1989). Cognitive–behavioral therapy and relationship therapy in the treatment of children referred for antisocial behavior. *Journal of Consulting and Clinical Psychology, 57,* 522–535.

Kazdin, A. E., Esveldt-Dawson, K., French, N. H., & Unis, A. S. (1987a). Effects of parent management training and problem-solving skills training combined in the treatment of antisocial child behavior. *Journal of the American Academy of Child and Adolescent Psychiatry, 26,* 416–424.

Kazdin, A. E., Esveldt-Dawson, K., French, N. H., & Unis, A. S. (1987b). Problem-solving skills training and relationship therapy in the treatment of antisocial child behavior. *Journal of Consulting and Clinical Psychology, 55,* 76–85.

Kazdin, A. E., French, N. H., Unis, A. S., & Esveldt-Dawson K. (1983). Assessment of childhood depression: Correspondence of child and parent ratings. *Journal of the American Academy of Child Psychiatry, 22,* 157–164.

Keller, C. E., & Lloyd, J. W. (1989). Cognitive training: Implications for arithmetic instruction. In J. N. Hughes & R. J. Hall (Eds.), *Cognitive-behavioral psychology in the schools: A comprehensive handbook* (pp. 280–304). New York: Guilford Press.

Kendall, P. C. (1977). On the efficacious use of verbal self-instructional procedures with children. *Cognitive Therapy and Research, 1,* 331–341.

Kendall, P. C. (1981a). Cognitive–behavioral interventions with children. In B. B. Lahey & A. E. Kazdin (Eds.), *Advances in clinical child psychology* (Vol. 4, pp. 53–90). New York: Plenum Press.

Kendall, P. C. (1981b). One-year follow-up of concrete versus conceptual cognitive–behavioral self-control training. *Journal of Consulting and Clinical Psychology, 49,* 748–749.

Kendall, P. C. (1982a). Cognitive processes and procedures in behavior therapy. In C. M. Franks, G. T. Wilson, P. C. Kendall, & K. D. Brownell, *Annual review of behavior therapy: Theory and practice* (Vol. 8, pp. 120–155). New York: Guilford Press.

Kendall, P. C. (1982b). Individual versus group cognitive–behavioral self-control training: One-year follow-up. *Behavior Therapy, 13,* 241–247.

Kendall, P. C. (1984). Social cognition and problem solving: A developmental and child–clinical interface. In B. Gholson & T. Rosenthal (Eds.), *Applications of cognitive–developmental theory* (pp. 115–148). New York: Academic Press.

Kendall, P. C. (1985). Toward a cognitive–behavioral model of child psychopathology and a critique of related interventions. *Journal of Abnormal Child Psychology, 13,* 357–372.

Kendall, P. C. (1989). The generalization and maintenance of behavior change: Comments, considerations and the "no-cure" criticism. *Behavior Therapy, 20,* 357–364.

Kendall, P. C. (1990). *Coping cat workbook.* (Available from Workbooks, 238 Meeting House Lane, Merion Station, PA 19066.)

Kendall, P. C. (Ed.). (1991a) *Child and adolescent therapy: Cognitive–behavioral procedures.* New York: Guilford Press.

Kendall, P. C. (1991b). Guiding theory for therapy with children and adolescents. In P. C. Kendall (Ed.), *Child and adolescent therapy: Cognitive–behavioral procedures* (pp. 3–22). New York: Guilford Press.

Kendall, P. C. (1992a). *Stop and think workbook* (2nd ed.). (Available from Workbooks, 238 Meeting House Lane, Merion Station, PA 19066.)

Kendall, P. C. (1992b). *Cognitive-behavioral therapy for impulsive children: Treatment manual* (2nd ed.). (Available from Workbooks, 238 Meeting House Lane, Merion Station, PA 19066.)

Kendall, P. C., & Bartel, N. R. (1990). *Teaching problem solving to students with learning and behavior problems: A manual for teachers.* (Available from Workbooks, 238 Meeting House Lane, Merion Station, PA 19066.)

Kendall, P. C., & Braswell, L. (1982a). Cognitive–behavioral assessment: Model, measures, and madness. In J. N. Butcher & C. D. Spielberger (Eds.), *Advances in personality assessment* (Vol. 1, pp. 35–82). Hillsdale, NJ: Erlbaum.

Kendall, P. C., & Braswell, L. (1982b). Cognitive–behavioral self-control therapy for children: A components analysis. *Journal of Consulting and Clinical Psychology, 50,* 672–689.

Kendall, P. C., & Braswell, L. (Producers). (1982c). *Cognitive behavioral self-control therapy for children* [videotape]. (Available from the first author, Department of Psychology, Weiss Hall, Temple University, Philadelphia, PA 19022.)

Kendall, P. C., & Braswell, L. (1985). *Cognitive–behavioral therapy for impulsive children* (1st ed.). New York: Guilford Press.

Kendall, P. C., & Brophy, C. (1981). Activity and attentional correlates of teacher ratings of hyperactivity. *Journal of Pediatric Psychology, 6,* 451–458.

Kendall, P. C., Cantwell, D., & Kazdin, A. E. (1989). Depression in children and adolescents: Assessment issues and recommendations. *Cognitive Therapy and Research, 13,* 109–146.

Kendall, P. C., Chansky, T. E., Kane, M., Kim, R., Kortlander, E., Ronan, K. R.,

Sessa, F., & Siqueland, L. (1992). *Anxiety disorder in youth: Cognitive–behavioral interventions.* Needham, MA: Allyn and Bacon.

Kendall, P. C., & Finch, A. J. Jr. (1976). A cognitive–behavioral treatment for impulsivity: A case study. *Journal of Consulting and Clinical Psychology, 44,* 852–857.

Kendall, P. C., & Finch, A. J. Jr. (1978). A cognitive–behavioral treatment for impulsivity: A group comparison study. *Journal of Consulting and Clinical Psychology, 46,* 110–118.

Kendall, P. C., & Finch, A. J. Jr. (1979). Developing nonimpulsive behavior in children: Cognitive–behavioral strategies for self-control: In P. C. Kendall & S. D. Hollon (Eds.), *Cognitive–behavioral interventions: Theory, research, and procedures* (pp. 37–80). New York: Academic Press.

Kendall, P. C., Finch, A. J., Little, V. L., Chirico, B. M., & Ollendick, T. H. (1978). Variations in a construct: Quantitative and qualitative differences in children's locus of control. *Journal of Consulting and Clinical Psychology, 46,* 590–592.

Kendall, P. C., & Fischler, G. L. (1984). Behavioral and adjustment correlates of problem solving: Validational analyses of interpersonal cognitive problem-solving measures. *Child Development, 55,* 879–892.

Kendall, P. C., & Grove, W., (1988). Normative comparison in therapy outcome. *Behavioral Assessment, 10,,* 147–158.

Kendall, P. C., & Hollon, S. D. (Eds.). (1979). *Cognitive–behavioral interventions: Theory, research, and procedures.* New York: Academic Press.

Kendall, P. C., & Ingram, R. (1989). Cognitive–behavioral perspectives: Theory and research on depression and anxiety. In P. C. Kendall & D. Watson (Eds.), *Anxiety and depression: Distinctive and overlapping features.* New York: Academic Press.

Kendall, P. C., & Korgeski, G. P. (1979). Assessment and cognitive–behavioral interventions. *Cognitive Therapy and Research, 3,* 1–21.

Kendall, P. C., & MacDonald, J. P. (in press). Cognition in the psychopathology of youth, and implications for treatment. In K. Dobson & P. C. Kendall (Eds.), *Psychopathology and cognition.* Orlando, FL: Academic Press.

Kendall, P. C., & Morris, R. J. (1991). Child therapy: Issues and recommendations. *Journal of Consulting and Clinical Psychology, 59,* 777–784.

Kendall, P. C., & Norton-Ford, J. D. (1982a). *Clinical psychology: Scientific and professional dimensions.* New York: Wiley.

Kendall, P. C., & Norton-Ford, J. D. (1982b). Therapy outcome research methods. In P. C. Kendall & J. N. Butcher (Eds.), *Handbook of research methods in clinical psychology* (pp. 429–460). New York: Wiley.

Kendall, P. C., Pellegrini, D., & Urbain, E. S. (1981a). Approaches to assessment for cognitive–behavioral interventions with children. In P. C. Kendall & S. D. Hollon (Eds.), *Assessment strategies for cognitive–behavioral interventions* (pp. 227–286). New York: Academic Press.

Kendall, P. C., & Reber, M., (1987). Reply to Abikoff and Gittelman's evaluation of cognitive training with medicated hyperactive children. *Archives of General Psychiatry, 8,* 77–79.

Kendall, P. C., Reber, M., McLeer, S., Epps, J., & Ronan, K. R. (1990). Cognitive–behavioral treatment of conduct-disordered children. *Cognitive Therapy and Research, 14,* 279–297.

Kendall, P. C., & Ronan, K. R. (1990). Assessment of children's anxieties, fears, and phobias: Cognitive–behavioral models and methods. In C. R. Reynolds & R. W. Kamphaus (Eds.), *Handbook of psychological and educational assessment of children: Personality, behavior, and context* (pp. 223–244). New York: Guilford Press.

Kendall, P. C., Ronan, K. R., & Epps, J. (1991). Aggression in children/adolescents: Cognitive–behavioral treatment perspectives (pp. 341–360). In D. Popler & K. Rubin (Eds.), *Development and treatment of childhood aggression.* Hillsdale, NJ: Erlbaum.

Kendall, P. C., & Sessa, F. M. (in press). Cognitive assessment for intervention. In T. R. Kratochwill & R. J. Morris (Eds.), *Handbook of psychotherapy with children.* Needham, MA: Allyn & Bacon.

Kendall, P. C., Vitousek, K. B., & Kane, M. (1992). Thought and action in psychotherapy: The cognitive–behavioral approaches. In M. Hersen, A. Kazdin., & A. Bellack (Eds.), *The clinical psychology handbook* (2nd ed., pp. 596–626). New York: Pergamon Press.

Kendall, P. C., & Wilcox, L. E. (1979). Self-control in children: Development of a rating scale. *Journal of Consulting and Clinical Psychology, 47,* 1020–1029.

Kendall, P. C., & Wilcox, L. E. (1980). A cognitive–behavioral treatment for impulsivity: Concrete versus conceptual training in non-self-controlled problem children. *Journal of Consulting and Clinical Psychology, 48,* 80–91.

Kendall, P. C., & Williams, C. L. (1986). Adolescent therapy: Treating the "marginal man." *Behavior Therapy, 17,* 522–537.

Kendall, P. C., & Zupan, B. A. (1981). Individual versus group application of cognitive–behavioral strategies for developing self-control in children. *Behavior Therapy, 12,* 344–359.

Kendall, P. C., Zupan, B. A., & Braswell, L. (1981b). Self-control in children: Further analyses of the Self-Control Rating Scale. *Behavior Therapy, 12,* 667–681.

Keogh, D. A., Whitman, T. L., & Maxwell, S. E. (1988). Self-instruction versus external instruction: Individual differences and training effectiveness. *Cognitive Therapy and Research, 12,* 591–610.

Kifer, R. E., Lewis, M. A., Green, D. R., & Phillips, E. L. (1974). Training pre-delinquent youths and their parents to negotiate conflict situations. *Journal of Applied Behavior Analysis, 7,* 357–364.

Kirmil-Gray, K., Duckham-Shoor, L., & Thoresen, C. E. (1980, November). *The effects of self-control instruction and behavior management training on the academic and social behavior of hyperactive children.* Paper presented at the meeting of the Association for Advancement of Behavior Therapy, New York.

Klein, N. C., Alexander, J. F., & Parsons, B. V. (1977). Impact of family systems intervention on recidivism and sibling delinquency: A model of primary prevention and program evaluation. *Journal of Consulting and Clinical Psychology, 45,* 469–474.

Kohlberg, L., Yaeger, J., & Hjentholm, E. (1968). Private speech: Four studies and a review of theories. *Child Development, 39,* 671–690.

Kolko, D. J., Loar, L. L., & Sturnick, D. (1990). Inpatient social–cognitive skills training groups with conduct-disordered and attention-deficit disordered children. *Journal of Child Psychology and Psychiatry, 31,* 737–748.

Kopel, S., & Arkowitz, H. (1975). The role of attribution and self-perception in behavior change: Implications for behavior therapy. *Genetic Psychology Monographs, 92,* 175–212.

Kopp, C. B. (1982). Antecedents of self-regulation: A developmental perspective. *Developmental Psychology, 18,* 199–214.

Krupski, A. (1986). Attention problems in youngsters with learning handicaps. In J. K. Torgeson & B. Y. L. Wong (Eds.), *Psychological and educational perspectives on learning disabilities* (pp. 161–192). New York: Academic Press.

Kuehne, C., Kehle, T. J., & McMahon, W. (1987). Differences between children with Attention Deficit Disorder, children with specific learning disabilities, and normal children. *Journal of School Psychology, 25,* 161–166

Kurdek, L. A. (1977). Structural components and intellectual correlates of cognitive perspective taking in first- through fourth-grade children. *Child Development, 48,* 1503–1511.

Kurdek, L. A., & Sinclair, R. J. (1988). Adjustment of young adolescents in two parent nuclear, stepfather, and mother- custody families. *Journal of Consulting and Clinical Psychology, 56,* 91–96.

Lahey, B. B., Green, K. D., & Forehand, R. (1980). On the independence of ratings of hyperactivity, conduct problems, and attentional deficit in children: A multiple regression analysis. *Journal of Consulting and Clinical Psychology, 48,* 566–574.

Lahey, B. B., Piacentini, J. C., McBurnett, K. Stone, P., Hartdagen, S., & Hynd, G. (1988). Psychopathology in the parents of children with conduct disorder and hyperactivity. *Journal of the American Academy of Child and Adolescent Psychiatry, 27,* 163–170.

Lahey, B. B., Stempniak, M., Robinson, E. J., & Tyroler, M. J. (1978). Hyperactivity and learning disabilities as independent dimensions of child behavior problems. *Journal of Abnormal Psychology, 87,* 333–340.

Lambert, N. M., Hartsough, C. S., Sassone, D., & Sandoval, J. (1987). Persistence of hyperactivity symptoms from childhood to adolescence and associated outcomes. *American Journal of Orthopsychiatry, 57,* 22–32.

Lambert, H. M., Sandoval, J., & Sassone, D. (1977, August). *Multiple prevalence estimates of hyperactivity in school children.* Paper presented at the meeting of the American Psychological Association, San Francisco, CA.

Larcen, S., Spivack, G., & Shure, M. B. (1972, April). *Problem-solving thinking and adjustment among dependent neglected pre-adolescents.* Paper presented at the meeting of the Eastern Psychological Association, Boston, MA.

Laufer, M. W., & Denhoff, C. (1957). Hyperkinetic behavior syndrome in children. *Journal of Pediatrics, 50,* 463–474.

Ledger, G. W., & Ryan, E. G. (1982). The effects of semantic integration training on recall for pictograph sentences. *Journal of Experimental Child Psychology, 33,* 39–54.

Ledwidge, B. (1978). Cognitive behavior modification: A step in the wrong direction? *Psychological Bulletin, 85*, 353–375.

Leon, J. A., & Pepe, H. J. (1983). Self-instructional training: Cognitive behavior modification for remediating arithmetic deficits. *Exceptional Children, 50*, 54–60.

Lobitz, G. K., & Johnson, S. M. (1975). Normal versus deviant children: A multimethod comparison. *Journal of Abnormal Child Psychology, 3*, 353–374.

Lochman, J. E. (1992). Cognitive–behavioral intervention with aggressive boys: Three-year follow-up and preventive effects. *Journal of Consulting and Clinical Psychology, 60*, 426–432.

Lochman, J. E., Burch, P. R., Curry, J. F., & Lampron, L B. (1984). Treatment and generalization effects of cognitive–behavioral and goal-setting interventions with aggressive boys. *Journal of Consulting and Clinical Psychology, 52*, 915–916.

Lochman, J. E., & Curry, J. F. (1986). Effects of social problem-solving training and self-instruction training with aggressive boys. *Journal of Clinical Child Psychology, 15*, 159–164.

Lochman, J. E., Lampron, L. B., Burch, P. R., & Curry, J. F. (1985). Client characteristics associated with behavior change for treated and untreated boys. *Journal of Abnormal Child Psychology, 13*, 527–538.

Lochman, J. E., Lampron, L. B., Gemmer, T. V., Harris, R., & Wyckoff, G. M. (1989). Teacher consultation and cognitive–behavioral interventions with aggressive boys. *Psychology in the Schools, 26*, 179–188.

Lochman, J. E., White, K. J., & Wayland, K. K. (1991). Cognitive–behavioral assessment and treatment with aggressive children. In P. C. Kendall (Ed.), *Child and adolescent therapy: Cognitive–behavioral procedures* (pp. 25–65). New York: Guilford Press.

Loeber, R. (1982). The stability of antisocial and delinquent behavior: A review. *Child Development, 53*, 1431–1446.

Loeber, R. (1985). Patterns and development of antisocial child behavior. In G. J. Whitehurst (Ed.), *Annals of child development* (Vol. 2). Greenwich, CT: JAI Press.

Loeber, R. (1989). Natural histories of juvenile conduct problems, substance use, and delinquency: Evidence for developmental progressions. In B. B. Lahey & A. E. Kazdin (Eds.), *Advances in clinical child psychology* (Vol. 11, pp. 73–124). New York: Plenum Press.

Loeber, R., Green, S., & Lahey, B. (1990). Mental health professionals' perception of the utility of children, mothers, and teachers as informants on childhood psychopathology. *Journal of Clinical Child Psychology, 19*, 136–143.

Loney, J., Comly, H. H., & Simon, B. (1975). Parental management, self-concept, and drug response in minimal brain dysfunction. *Journal of Learning Disabilities, 8*, 187–190.

Loney, J., & Milich, R. (1982). Hyperactivity, inattention, and aggression in clinical practice. In D. Routh & M. Wolraich (Ed.), *Advances in developmental and behavioral pediatrics* (Vol. 3, pp. 113–147). Greenwich, CT: JAI Press.

Loper, A. B. (1980). Metacognitive development: Implications for cognitive training. *Exceptional Education Quarterly, 1,* 1–8.

Lorber, N. M. (1970). The Ohio Social Acceptance Scale. *Educational Research, 12,* 240–243.

Lovaas, O. I. (1964). Cue properties of words: The control of operant responding by rate and content of verbal operants. *Child Development, 35,* 245–256.

Luk, S. L. (1985). Direct observation studies of hyperactive behaviors. *Journal of the American Academy of Child Psychiatry, 24,* 338–344.

Luria, A. R. (1959). The directive function of speech in development and dissolution. *Word, 15,* 341–352.

Luria, A. R. (1961). *The role of speech in the regulation of normal and abnormal behaviors.* New York: Liveright.

Lytton, H. (1976). The socialization of two-year-old boys: Ecological findings. *Journal of Child Psychology and Psychiatry, 17,* 287–304.

MacFarlane, J., Allen, L., & Honzik, M. (1954). *A developmental study of the behavior problems of normal children between 21 months and 14 years.* Berkeley, CA: University of California Press.

Mahoney, M. J. (1977a). Personal science: A cognitive learning therapy. In A. Ellis & R. Grieger (Eds.), *Handbook of rational psychotherapy* (pp. 352–366). New York: Springer.

Mahoney, M. J. (1977b). Reflections on the cognitive–learning trend in psychotherapy. *American Psychologist, 32,* 5–13.

Mahoney, M. J., & Arnkoff, D. B. (1978). Cognitive and self-control therapies. In S. L. Garfield & A. E. Bergin (Eds.), *Handbook of psychotherapy and behavior change* (2nd ed., pp. 689–721). New York: Wiley.

Mannuzza, S., & Klein, R. (1987). *Schedule for the Assessment of Conduct, Hyperactivity, Anxiety, Mood, and Psychoactive Substances (CHAMPS).* Children's Behavior Disorder Clinic, Long Island Jewish Medical Center, New Hyde Park, NY 11042.

Marlatt, G. A. (1979). Alcohol use and problem drinking: A cognitive–behavioral analysis. In P. C. Kendall & S. D. Hollon (Eds.), *Cognitive–behavioral interventions: Theory, research, and procedures* (pp. 319–356). New York: Academic Press.

Mash, E. J., & Terdal, L. G. (Eds.). (1988). *Behavioral assessment of childhood disorders* (2nd ed.) New York: Guilford Press.

Mash, E. J., Terdal, L., & Anderson, K. (1973). The response-class matrix: A procedure for recording parent child interactions. *Journal of Consulting and Clinical Psychology, 40,* 163–164.

McClure, L. F., Chinsky, J. M., & Larcen, S. W. (1978). Enhancing social problem-solving performance in an elementary school setting. *Journal of Educational Psychology, 70,* 504–513.

McCord, W., McCord, J., & Gudeman, J. (1960). *Origins of alcoholism.* Palo Alto, CA: Stanford University Press.

McGee, R., Williams, S., & Silva, P. A. (1985). Factor structure and correlates of ratings on inattention, hyperactivity, and antisocial behavior in a large sample of 9-year-old children from the general population. *Journal of Consulting and Clinical Psychology, 53,* 480–490.

McMahon, R. J., & Forehand, R. (1988). Conduct disorders. In E. J. Mash & L. G. Terdal (Eds.), *Behavioral assessment of childhood disorders* (2nd ed., pp. 105–153). New York: Guilford Press.

McMahon, R. J., & Wells, K. C. (1989). Conduct disorders. In E. J. Mash & R. A. Barkley (Eds.) *Treatment of childhood disorders* (pp. 73–132). New York: Guilford Press.

Meacham, J. A. (1978). Verbal guidance through remembering the goals of action. *Child Development, 49,* 188–193.

Mednick, S. A. (1975). Autonomic nervous system recovery and psychopathology. *Scandinavian Journal of Behavior Therapy, 4,* 55–68.

Meichenbaum, D. H. (1971). Examination of model characteristics in reducing avoidance behavior. *Journal of Personality and Social Psychology, 17,* 298–307.

Meichenbaum, D. H. (1975). Self-instructional methods. In F. Kanfer & A. Goldstein (Eds.), *Helping people change* (pp. 357–391). New York: Pergamon Press.

Meichenbaum, D. H. (1976b). Toward a cognitive theory of self-control. In G. Schwartz & D. Shapiro (Eds.), *Consciousness and self-regulation* (Vol. 1, pp. 223–260). New York: Plenum Press.

Meichenbaum, D. H. (1977). *Cognitive–behavior modification: An integrative approach.* New York: Plenum Press.

Meichenbaum, D. H. (1979b). Teaching children self-control. In B. B. Lahey & A. E. Kazdin (Eds.), *Advances in clinical child psychology* (Vol. 2, pp. 1–35). New York: Plenum Press.

Meichenbaum, D. H. (1985). *Stress inoculation training.* New York: Pergamon Press.

Meichenbaum, D. H., & Goodman, J. (1971). Training impulsive children to talk to themselves: A means of developing self-control. *Journal of Abnormal Psychology, 77,* 115–126.

Mendelson, N., Johnson, N., & Stewart, M. (1971). Hyperactive children as teenagers: A follow-up study. *Journal of Nervous and Mental Diseases, 153,* 272–279.

Messer, S. B. (1976). Reflection impulsivity: A review. *Psychological Bulletin, 83,* 1026–1052.

Meyers, J., & Yelich, G. (1989). Cognitive–behavioral approaches in psychoeducational consultation. In J. N. Hughes & R. J. Hall (Eds.), *Cognitive–behavioral psychology in the schools: A comprehensive handbook* (pp. 501–534). New York: Guilford Press.

Milich, R., & Fitzgerald, G. (1985). Validation of inattention/overactivity and aggression ratings with classroom observation. *Journal of Consulting and Clinical Psychology, 53,* 139–140.

Milich, R., & Kramer, J. (1984). Reflections on impulsivity: An empirical investigation of impulsivity as a construct. In K. Gadow (Ed.), *Advances in learning and behavioral disabilities* (Vol. 3, pp. 57–94). Greenwich, CT: JAI Press.

Milich, R. S., Loney, J., & Landau, S. (1982). Independent dimensions of hyperactivity and aggression: A validation with playroom observation data. *Journal of Abnormal Psychology, 91,* 183–198.

Miller, L. C., Hampe, E., Barrett, C., & Noble, H. (1971). Children's deviant behavior within the general population. *Journal of Consulting and Clinical Psychology, 37,* 16–22.

Minde, K., Lewin, D., Weiss, G., Lavigueur, H., Douglas, V. I., & Sykes, E. (1971). The hyperactive child in elementary school: A five-year controlled follow-up. *Exceptional Children, 38,* 215–227.

Minde, K., Weiss, G., & Mendelson, N. (1972). A five-year follow-up study of 91 hyperactive schoolchildren. *Journal of American Academy of Child Psychiatry, 11,* 595–610.

Mischel, W. (1974). Processes in delay of gratification. In L. Berkowitz (Ed.), *Advances in experimental social psychology* (Vol. 7, pp. 249–292). New York: Academic Press.

Mischel, W., & Patterson, C. J. (1976). Substantive and structural elements of effective plans for self-control. *Journal of Personality and Social Psychology, 34,* 942–950.

Monohan, J., & O'Leary, K. D. (1971). Effects of self-instruction on rule-breaking behavior. *Psychological Reports, 29,* 1051–1066.

Montague, M., & Bos, C. S., (1986). The effect of cognitive strategy training on verbal math problem-solving performance of learning-disabled adolescents. *Journal of Learning Disabilities, 19,* 26–33.

Moon, C. E., & Marlowe, M. (1987). Construct validity of the Walker Problem Behavior Identification Checklist. *Educational and Psychological Measurement, 47,* 249–252.

Mussen, P. H. (1963). *The psychological development of the child.* Englewood Cliffs, NJ: Prentice-Hall.

Myers, P. I., & Hammil, D. D. (1990). *Learning disabilities: Basic concepts, assessment practices, and instructional strategies* (4th ed.). Austin, TX: Pro-Ed.

Nay, W. R. (1986). Analogue measures. In A. R. Ciminero, K. S. Calhoun, & H. E. Adams (Eds.), *Handbook of behavioral assessment* (2nd ed., pp. 223–252). New York: Wiley.

Neilans, T. H., & Israel, A. C. (1981) Towards maintenance and generalization of behavior change: Teaching children self-regulation and self-instructional skills. *Cognitive Therapy and Research, 5,* 189–196.

Nelson, W., & Birkimer, J. C. (1978). Role of self-instruction and self-reinforcement in the modification of impulsivity. *Journal of Consulting and Clinical Psychology, 46,* 183.

Nezu, A., Nezu, C., & Perri, M. (1989). *Problem-solving therapy for depression: Theory, research, and clinical guidelines.* New York: Wiley.

Nowicki, S. Jr., & Strickland, B. R. (1973). A locus-of-control scale for children. *Journal of Consulting and Clinical Psychology, 40,* 148–154.

Nye, F. I. (1958). *Family relationships and delinquent behavior.* New York: Wiley.

O'Leary, K. D. (1968). The effects of self-instruction on immoral behavior. *Journal of Experimental Child Psychology, 6,* 297–301.

Palinscar, A., & Brown, A. L. (1984). Reciprocal teaching of comprehension-fostering and comprehension-monitoring activities. *Cognition and Instruction, 1,* 117–175.

Palkes, H., Stewart, M., & Freedman, J. (1972). Improvement in maze performance of hyperactive boys as a function of verbal-training procedures. *Journal of Special Education, 5,* 337–342.

Palkes, H., Stewart, M., & Kahana, B. (1968). Porteus maze performance of hyperactive boys after training in self-directed verbal commands. *Child Development, 39,* 817–826.

Parry, P. (1973). *The effect of reward on the performance of hyperactive children.* Unpublished doctoral dissertation, McGill University, Montreal.

Parsons, B. V., & Alexander, J. F. (1973). Short-term family intervention: A therapy outcome study. *Journal of Consulting and Clinical Psychology, 41,* 195–201.

Parsons, J. A. (1972). The reciprocal modification of arithmetic behavior and program development. In G. Semb (Ed.), *Behavior analysis and education—1972* (pp. 185–199). Lawrence, KS: University of Kansas Department of Human Development.

Paternite, C. E., Loney, J., & Langhorne, J. E., Jr. (1976). Relationships between symptomatology and SES-related factors in hyperkinetic/MBD boys. *American Journal of Orthopsychiatry, 46,* 291–301.

Patterson, C., & Mischel, W. (1976). Effects of temptation-inhibiting and task-facilitating plans on self-control. *Journal of Personality and Social Psychology, 33,* 207–217.

Patterson, G. R. (1976). The aggressive child: Victim and architect of a coercive system. In E. J. Mash, L. Hamerlynck, & L. Handy (Eds.), *Behavior modification and families: I. Theory and research* (pp. 267–316). New York: Brunner/Mazel.

Patterson, G. R., & Bank, L. (1989). Some amplifying mechanisms for pathologic processes in families. In M. Gunnar (Ed.), *Minnesota symposium in child development* (pp. 167–209). Englewood Cliffs, NJ: LEA.

Patterson, G. R., Ray, R. S., Shaw, D. A., & Cobb, J. A. (1969). *Manual for coding of interactions.* (1969 rev.). New York: Microfiche.

Patterson, G. R., Reid, J. B., Jones, R. R., & Conger, R. E. (1975). *A social learning approach to family intervention: Families with aggressive children* (Vol. 1). Eugene, OR: Castalia.

Paulauskas, S. L., & Campbell, S. B. G. (1979). Social perspective-taking and teacher ratings of peer interaction in hyperactive boys. *Journal of Abnormal Child Psychology, 7,* 483–494.

Pelham, W. E., & Bender, M. E. (1982). Peer relationships in hyperactive children: Description and treatment. In K. D. Gadow & I. Bialer (Eds.), *Advances in learning and behavioral disabilities* (Vol. 1, pp. 365–346). Greenwich, CT: JAI Press.

Pelham, W. E., Carlson, C., Sams, S., Vallano, G., Dixon, M. J., & Hoza, B. (in press). Separate and combined effects of methylphenidate and behavior modification on classroom behavior and academic performance of ADHD boys: Group effects and individual differences. *Journal of Consulting and Clinical Psychology.*

Pelham, W. E., Milich, R. Murphy, D., & Murphy, H. (1989). Normative data on the IOWA Conners Teacher Rating Scale. *Journal of Clinical Child Psychology, 18,* 259–262.

Pellegrini, D. S. (1980). *The social–cognitive qualities of stress-resistant children*. Unpublished doctoral dissertation, University of Minnesota.

Pfiffner, L. J., Jouriles, E. N., Brown, M. M., Etscheidt, M. A., & Kelly, J. A. (1990). Effects of problem-solving therapy on outcomes of parent training for single-parent families. *Child and Family Behavior Therapy, 12,* 1–11.

Phares, V. Compas, B. E. & Howell, D. (1989). Perspectives on child behavior problems: Comparisons of children's self-reports with parent and teacher reports. *Psychological Assessment: A Journal of Consulting and Clinical Psychology, 1,* 68–71.

Piaget, G. W. (1972). Training parents to communicate. In A. A. Lazarus (Ed.), *Clinical behavior therapy* (pp. 155–173). New York: Brunner/Mazel.

Piaget, J. (1926). *The language and thought of the child.* New York: Harcourt-Brace.

Piers, E. V., & Harris, D. B. (1969). *The Piers–Harris Children's Self-Concept Scale.* Nashville: Counselor Recordings and Tests.

Pisterman, S., McGrath, P., Firestone, P., Goodman, J. T., Webster, I., & Mallory, R. (1989). Outcome of parent-mediated treatment of preschoolers with attention deficit disorder with hyperactivity. *Journal of Consulting and Clinical Psychology, 57,* 628–635.

Platt, J. J., & Spivack, G. (1972a). Problem-solving thinking of psychiatric patients. *Journal of Consulting and Clinical Psychology, 39,* 148–151.

Platt, J. J., & Spivack, G. (1972b). Social competence and effective problem-solving thinking in psychiatric patients. *Journal of Clinical Psychology, 28,* 3–5.

Platt, J. J., & Spivack, G. (1973). Studies in problem-solving thinking of psychiatric patients: Patient control differences and factorial structure of problem-solving thinking. *Proceedings, of the 81st Annual Convention of the American Psychological Association, 8,* 461–462.

Platt, J. J., Spivack, G., Altman, N., Altman, D., & Peizer, S. B. (1974). Adolescent problem-solving thinking. *Journal of Consulting and Clinical Psychology, 42,* 787–793.

Porter, J. E., & Rourke, B. P. (1985). Socioemotional functioning of learning-disabled children: A subtypal analysis of personality patterns. In B. P. Rourke (Ed.), *Neuropsychology of learning disabilities: Essentials of subtype analysis* (pp. 257–280). New York: Guilford Press.

Porteus, S. D. (1933). *The maze test and mental differences.* Vineland, NJ: Smith.

Porteus, S. D. (1955). *The maze test: Recent advances.* Palo Alto, CA: Pacific Books.

Pressley, M., & Levin, J. R. (1986). Elaborative learning strategies for the inefficient learner. In S. J. Ceci (Ed.), *Handbook of cognitive, social and neuropsychological aspects of learning disabilities* (pp. 175–211). Hillsdale, NJ: Erlbaum.

Prior, M., & Sanson, A. (1986). Attention-deficit disorder with hyperactivity: A critique. *Journal of Child Psychology and Psychiatry, 27,* 307–312.

Puig-Antich, J. & Chambers, W. (1978). *Schedule for Affective Disorders and Schizophrenia for School-aged Children.* New York: New York State Psychiatric Institute.

Quay, H. C., & Peterson, D. R. (1983). *Interim manual for the Revised Behavior Problem Checklist.* Unpublished manuscript, University of Miami.

Rapoport, J. L., Quinn, P. O., Burg, C., & Bartley, L. (1979). Can hyperactivities be identified in infancy? In R. L. Trites (Ed.), *Hyperactivity in children: Etiology, measurement, and treatment implications* (pp. 103–115). Baltimore, MD: University Park.

Rapport, M. D., Jones, J. T., DuPaul, G. J., Kelly, K. L., Gardner, M. J., Tucker, S. B., & Shea, M. S. (1987). Attention-deficit disorder and methylphenidate: Group and single-subject analyses of dose effects on attention in clinic and classroom settings . *Journal of Clinical Child Psychology, 16,* 329–338.

Rapport, M. D., Stoner, G., DuPaul, G. J., Kelly, K. L., Tucker, S. B., & Schoeler, T. (1988). Attention-deficit disorder and methylphenidate: A multilevel analysis of dose-response effects on children's impulsivity across settings. *Journal of the American Academy of Child and Adolescent Psychiatry, 27,* 60–69.

Reeves, J. C., Werry, J. S., Elkind, G. S., & Zametkin, A. (1987). Attention deficit, conduct, oppositional and anxiety disorders in children. II. Clinical characteristics. *Journal of the American Academy of Child and Adolescent Psychiatry, 26,* 144–155.

Reid, M. K., & Borkowski, J. G. (1987). Causal attributions of hyperactive children: Implications for teaching strategies and self-control. *Journal of Educational Psychology, 79,* 296–307.

Reynolds, W., & Stark, K. D. (1986). Self-control in children: A multimethod examination of treatment outcome measures. *Journal of Abnormal Child Psychology, 14,* 13–23.

Richard, B. A., & Dodge, K. A. (1982). Social maladjustment and problem-solving in school-aged children. *Journal of Consulting and Clinical Psychology, 50,* 226–233.

Rickel, A., Eshelman, A. K., & Loigman, G. A. (1983). Social problem solving training: A follow-up study of cognitive and behavioral effects. *Journal of Abnormal Child Psychology, 11,* 15–28.

Riddle, M., & Roberts, A. H. (1974). *The Porteus Mazes: A critical evaluation* (Report No. PR-74-3). Minneapolis, MN: University of Minnesota, Department of Psychiatry.

Riddle, M., & Roberts, A. H. (1977). Delinquency, delay of gratification, recidivism, and the Porteus Maze tests. *Psychological Bulletin, 84,* 417–425.

Roberts, M. A. (1990). A behavioral observation method for differentiating hyperactive and aggressive boys. *Journal of Abnormal Child Psychology, 2,* 131–142.

Roberts, M. A., Milich, R., & Loney, J. (1985). *Structured Observations of Academic and Play Setting (SOAPS): Manual.* (Available from Mary Ann Roberts, PhD, Psychology, Hospital School, University of Iowa, Iowa City, IA 52242.)

Roberts, M. A., Milich, R., Loney, J., & Caputo, J. (1981). A multitrait multimethod analysis of variance of teachers' ratings of aggression, hyperactivity, and inattention. *Journal of Abnormal Child Psychology, 9,* 371–380.

Roberts, M. A., Ray, R. S., & Roberts, R. J. (1984). A playroom observational procedure for assessing hyperactive boys. *Journal of Pediatric Psychology, 9,* 177–191.

Robin, A. L., Fischel, J. E., & Brown, K. E. (1984). The measurement of self-control in children: Validation of the Self-Control Rating Scale. *Journal of Pediatric Psychology, 9,* 165–175.

Robin, A. L., & Foster, S. L. (1989). *Negotiating parent–adolescent conflict: A behavioral–family systems approach.* New York: Guilford Press.

Robin, A. L., Kent, R., O'Leary, K. D., Foster, S., & Prinz, R. (1977). An approach to teaching parents and adolescents problem-solving communication skills: A preliminary report. *Behavior Therapy, 8,* 639–643.

Robins, L. (1966). *Deviant children grow up.* Baltimore, MD: Williams & Wilkins.

Roff, M. (1961). Childhood social interactions and young adult bad conduct. *Journal of Abnormal and Social Psychology, 63,* 333–337.

Roff, M., Sells, S. S., & Golden, M. M. (1972). *Social adjustment and personality development in children.* Minneapolis, MN: University of Minnesota Press.

Rondal, J. (1976). Investigation of the regulatory power of impulsive and meaningful aspects of speech. *Genetic Psychology Monographs, 94,* 3–33.

Rosenthal, T., & Bandura, A. (1978). Psychological modeling: Theory and practice. In S. L. Garfield & A. E. Bergin (Eds.), *Handbook of psychotherapy and behavior change* (2nd ed, pp. 621–658). New York: Wiley.

Ross, D. M., & Ross, S. A. (1976). *Hyperactivity: Research, theory, and action.* New York: Wiley.

Rotter, J. B. (1966). Generalized expectancies for internal versus external control of reinforcement. *Psychological Monographs, 30* (Whole No. 1).

Rotter, J. B., & Hochreich, D. J. (1975). *Personality.* Glenview, IL: Scott, Foresman.

Routh, D. K. (1980). Developmental aspects of hyperactivity. In C. K. Whalen & B. Henker (Eds.), *Hyperactive children: The social ecology of identification and treatment* (pp. 55–71). New York: Academic Press.

Rubin, K., & Krasnor, L. (1984). Social cognitive and social behavioral perspectives on problem solving. In M. Perlmutter (Ed.), *Social cognition: Minnesota Symposium on Child Psychology* (Vol. 18, pp. 1–68). Hillsdale, NJ: Erlbaum.

Rutter, M. (1974). Epidemiological and conceptual considerations in risk research. In E. J. Anthony & C. Koupernik (Eds.), *The child in his family: Children at psychiatric risk* (pp. 167–179). New York: Wiley.

Rutter, M., Cox, A., Tupling, C., Berger, M., & Yule, W. (1975). Attainment and adjustment in two geographical areas: I. Prevalence of psychiatric disorders. *British Journal of Psychiatry, 126,* 493–509.

Rutter, M., Tizard, J., Yule, W., Graham, P., & Whitmore, K. (1976). Research report: Isle of Wight studies, 1964–1974. *Psychological Medicine, 6,* 313–332.

Ryan, E. B., Ledger, G. W., & Robine, D. M. (1984). Effects of semantic integration training on the recall for pictograph sentences by kindergarten and first-grade children. *Journal of Educational Psychology, 76,* 371–382.

Ryan, E. B., Weed, K. A., & Short, E. J. (1986). Cognitive behavior modification: Promoting active, self-regulatory learning styles. In J. K. Torgesen & B. Y. L. Wong (Eds.), *Psychological and educational perspective on learning disabilities* (pp. 367–397). New York: Academic Press.

Safer, D. J., & Allen, R. P. (1976). *Hyperactive children: Diagnosis and management.* Baltimore, MD: University Park.

Salkind, N. J. (1979). *The development of norms for the Matching Familiar Figures test.* Manuscript available from the author, University of Kansas.

Sameroff, A. J. (1987). Transactional risk factors and prevention. In J. A. Steinberg & M. M. Silverstein (Eds.), *Preventing mental disorders: A research perspective* (pp. 74–89). Rockville, MD: U. S. Department of Health and Human Services.

Sanders, L. W. (1962). Issues in early mother–child interaction. *Journal of the American Academy of Child Psychiatry, 1,* 141–166.

Sarason, I. G. (1968). Verbal learning, modeling and juvenile delinquency. *American Psychologist, 23,* 254–266.

Sarason, I. G. (1975). Test anxiety and the self-disclosing model. *Journal of Consulting and Clinical Psychology, 43,* 148–153.

Sarason, I. G., & Ganzer, V. J. (1973). Modeling and group discussion in the rehabilitation of juvenile delinquents. *Journal of Counseling Psychology, 20,* 442–449.

Sarason, I. G., & Sarason, B. R. (1981). Teaching cognitive and social skills to high school students. *Journal of Consulting and Clinical Psychology, 49,* 908–918.

Schachar, R., Taylor, E., Wieselberg, M., Thorley, G., & Rutter, M. (1987). Changes in family function and relationships in children who respond to methylphenidate. *Journal of the American Academy of Child and Adolescent Psychiatry, 26,* 728–732.

Schachar, R., & Wachsmuth, R. (1990). Hyperactivity and parental psychopathology. *Journal of Child Psychology and Psychiatry, 31,* 381–392.

Schallow, J. R. (1975). Locus of control and success at self-modification. *Behavior Therapy, 6,* 667–671.

Schleifer, M., Weiss, G., Cohen, N., Elman, M., Cvejic, H., & Kruger, E. (1975). Hyperactivity in preschoolers and the effect of methylphenidate. *American Journal of Orthopsychiatry, 45,* 38–50.

Schleser, R., Meyers, A., & Cohen, R. (1981). Generalization of self-instructions: Effects of general versus specific content, active rehearsal, and cognitive level. *Child Development, 52,* 335–340.

Schunk, D. H. (1982). Effects of effort attributional feedback on children's perceived self-efficacy and achievement. *Journal of Educational Psychology, 74,* 548–556.

Selman, R. L. (1980). *The growth of interpersonal understanding: Developmental and clinical analyses.* New York: Academic Press.

Selman, R. L., Beardslee, W., Schultz, L. H., Krupa, M., & Poderefsky, D. (1986). Assessing adolescent interpersonal negotiation strategies: Toward the integration of structural and functional models. *Developmental Psychology, 22,* 450–459.

Selman, R. L., & Jaquette, D. (1978). Stability and oscillation in interpersonal awareness: A clinical developmental analysis. In C. B. Keasey (Ed.), *The XXVth Nebraska Symposium on Motivation.* Lincoln, NE: University of Nebraska Press.

Selman, R. L., Jaquette, D., & Lavin, R. (1977). Interpersonal awareness in children: Toward an integration of developmental and clinical child psychology. *American Journal of Orthopsychiatry, 47,* 264–274.

Sharp, K. C. (1981). Impact of interpersonal problem-solving training on preschoolers' social competency. *Journal of Applied Developmental Psychology, 2,* 129–143.

Shaw, D. S., & Emery, R. B. (1988). Chronic family adversity and school-age children's adjustment. *Journal of the American Academy of Child and Adolescent Psychiatry, 27,* 200–206.

Shure, M. B., & Spivack, G. (1970). *Problem-solving capacity, social class and adjustment among nursery school children.* Paper presented at the meeting of the Eastern Psychological Association, Atlantic City, NJ.

Shure, M. B., & Spivack, G. (1972). Means–end thinking, adjustment and social class among elementary school-aged children. *Journal of Consulting and Clinical Psychology, 38,* 348–353.

Shure, M. B., & Spivack, G. (1978). *Problem-solving techniques in childrearing.* San Francisco: Jossey-Bass.

Shure, M. B., Spivack, G., & Jaeger, M. (1971). Problem-solving thinking and adjustment among disadvantaged preschool children. *Child Development, 42,* 1791–1803.

Silver, A. A., & Hagin, R. A. (1990). *Disorders of learning in childhood.* New York: Wiley.

Spaccarelli, S., Cotler, S., & Penman, D. (1992). Problem- solving skills training as a supplement to behavioral parent training. *Cognitive Therapy and Research, 16,* 1–18.

Speedie, S. M., Houtz, J., Ringenbach, S., & Feldhusen, J. (1973). Abilities measured by the Purdue Elementary Problem-Solving Inventory. *Psychological Reports, 33,* 959–963.

Spivack, G., Haimes, P. E., & Spotts, J. (1967). *Devereux Adolescent Behavior Rating Scale.* Devon, PA: Devereux Foundation.

Spivack, G., & Levine, M. (1963). *Self-regulation in acting-out and normal adolescents* (Report No. M-4531). Washington, DC: National Institute of Mental Health.

Spivack, G., Platt, J. J., & Shure, M. B. (1976). *The problem-solving approach to adjustment.* San Francisco: Jossey-Bass.

Spivack, G., & Shure, M. B. (1974). *Social adjustment of young children: A cognitive approach to solving real-life problems.* San Francisco: Jossey-Bass.

Spivack, G., & Swift, M. (1973). The classroom behavior of children: A critical review of teacher-administered rating scales. *Journal of Special Education, 7,* 55–89.

Stark, K. D., Rouse, L. W., & Livingston, R. (1991). Treatment of depression during childhood and adolescence: Cognitive-behavioral procedures for individual and family. In P. C. Kendall (Ed.), *Child and adolescent therapy: Cognitive–behavioral procedures* (pp. 165–206). New York: Guilford Press.

Stoff, D., Friedman, E., Pollock, L., Vitiello, B., Kendall, P. C., & Bridger, W. (1989). Elevated platelet MAO is related to impulsivity in disruptive behavior disorders. *Journal of the American Academy of Child and Adolescent Psychiatry, 28,* 754–760.

Stokes, T. F., & Osnes, P. G. (1989). An operant pursuit of generalization. *Behavior Therapy, 20,* 337–355.

Stone, G., Hinds, W., & Schmidt, G. (1975). Teaching mental health behaviors to elementary school children. *Professional Psychology, 6,* 34–40.

Sturge, C. (1982). Reading retardation and antisocial behaviour. *Journal of Child Psychology and Psychiatry, 23,* 21–31.

Swanson, H. L. (Ed.). (1991). *Handbook on the assessment of learning disabilities: Theory, research, and practice.* Austin, TX: Pro-Ed.

Swanson, J. M. (1985). Measures of cognitive functioning appropriate for use in pediatric psychopharmacology research. *Psychopharmacology Bulletin, 21,* 887–890.

Szatmari, P., Offord, D. R., & Boyle, M. H. (1989). Correlates-associated impairments, and patterns of service utilization of children with attention-deficit disorders: Findings from the Ontario child health study. *Journal of Child Psychology and Psychiatry, 30,* 205–217.

Tant, J. L. (1978). *Problem-solving in hyperactive and reading-disabled boys.* Unpublished doctoral dissertation, McGill University.

Taylor, H. G. (1988). Learning disabilities. In E. J. Mash & L. G. Terdal (Eds.), *Behavioral assessment of childhood disorders* (2nd ed., pp. 402–450). New York: Guilford Press.

Taylor, H. G. (1989). Learning disabilities. In E. J. Mash & R. A. Barkley (Eds.), *Treatment of childhood disorders* (pp. 347–380). New York: Guilford Press.

Thackwray, D., Meyers, A., Schleser, R., & Cohen, R. (1985). Achieving generalization with general versus specific self-instructions: Effects on academically deficient children. *Cognitive Therapy and Research, 9,* 297–308.

Thomas, A., Chess, S., & Birch, H. G. (1968). *Temperament and behavior disorders in children.* New York: New York University Press.

Tolman, E. C. (1932). *Purposive behavior in animals and men.* New York: Century.

Tolman, E. C. (1951). *Collected papers in psychology.* Reprinted as *Behavior and psychological man.* Berkeley, CA: University of California Press.

Trites, R. L. (Ed.) (1979). *Hyperactivity in children: Etiology, measurement, and treatment implications.* Baltimore, MD: University Park.

Trites, R. L., Dugas, E., Lynch, G., & Ferguson, H. B. (1979). Prevalence of hyperactivity. *Journal of Pediatric Psychology, 4,* 179–188.

Turkewitz, H., O'Leary, K. D., & Ironsmith, M. (1975). Generalization and maintenance of appropriate behavior through self-control. *Journal of Consulting and Clinical Psychology, 43,* 577–583.

Ullmann, R. K., Sleator, E. K., & Sprague, R. L. (1985). A change of mind: The Conners Abbreviated Rating Scales reconsidered. *Journal of Abnormal Child Psychology, 13,* 553–565.

U.S. Department of Education. (1988). *Tenth annual report to Congress on the implementation of PL94-142.* Washington, DC: U.S. Government Printing Office.

U. S. Department of Education. (1991, September). *Memorandum on the subject of clarification of policy to address the needs of children with Attention Deficit Disorder with general and/or special education.* Washington, DC: Author.

U. S. Public Law 94-142 (The Education for All Handicapped Children Act). (1977, December 29). *Federal Register* (pp. 65,082–65,085).

Urbain, E. S. (1979). *Interpersonal problem-solving training and social perspective-taking training with impulsive children via modeling role-play and self-instruction.* Unpublished doctoral dissertation, University of Minnesota.

Urbain, E. S. (1982). *Social skills training workshop and friendship group manual.* St. Paul, MN: Wilder Child Guidance Center.

Urbain, E. S. (1985). *Friendship group manual (elementary grades) (Interpersonal problem-solving training for friendship-making)*. St. Paul, MN: Wilder Child Guidance Center.

Urbain, E. S., & Kendall, P. C. (1980). Review of social-cognitive problem-solving interventions with children. *Psychological Bulletin, 88,* 109–143.

Urbain, E. S., & Kendall, P. C. (1981). *Interpersonal problem-solving, social perspective-taking, and behavioral contingencies: A comparison of group approaches with impulsive-aggressive children*. Unpublished manuscript, University of Minnesota.

Urbain, E. S., & Savage, P. (1989). Interpersonal cognitive problem-solving training with children in the schools. In J. Hughes & R. Hall (Eds.,) *Cognitive–behavioral psychology in the schools: A comprehensive handbook*. New York: Guilford Press.

Varni, J. W., & Henker, B. (1979). A self-regulation approach to the treatment of three hyperactive boys. *Child Behavior Therapy, 1,* 171–191.

Vitiello, B., Stoff, D., Atkins, M., & Mahoney, A. (1990). Soft neurological signs and impulsivity in children. *Journal of Developmental and Behavioral Pediatrics, 11,* 112–115.

Vygotsky, L. S. (1962). *Thought and language*. New York: Wiley.

Vygotsky, L. S. (1978). *Mind in society*. Cambridge, MA: Harvard University Press. (Original works published 1930, 1933, and 1935)

Vygotsky, L. S. (1987). Thinking and speech. In *The collected works of L. S. Vygotsky: Vol. 1. Problems of general psychology* (N. Minick, Trans.). New York: Plenum Press. (Original work published 1934)

Wagner, I. (1975, April 1). *Reflection-impulsivity re-examined: Analysis and modification of cognitive strategies*. Paper presented at the Biennial Meeting of the Society for Research in Child Development, Denver.

Wahler, R. G., House, A. E., & Stambaugh, E. E. (1976). *Ecological assessment of child problem behavior*. New York: Pergamon Press.

Walczyk, J. J. & Hall, V. C. (1989). Is the failure to monitor comprehension an instance of cognitive impulsivity? *Journal of Educational Psychology, 81,* 294–298.

Walker, H. M. (1970). *The Walker Problem Behavior Identification Checklist*. Los Angeles: Psychological Services.

Wechsler, D. (1949). *Wechsler Intelligence Scale for Children*. New York: Psychological Corp.

Weiss, G. (1975). A natural history of hyperactivity in childhood and treatment with stimulant medication at different ages: A summary of research findings. *International Journal of Mental Health, 4,* 213–226.

Weiss, G., & Hechtman, L. T. (1986). *Hyperactive children grown up: Empirical findings and theoretical considerations*. New York: Guilford Press.

Weiss, G., Minde, K., Werry, J. S., Douglas, V. I., & Nemeth, E. (1971). Studies on the hyperactive child. VIII: Five-year follow-up. *Archives of General Psychiatry, 24,* 409–414.

Weissberg, R. P., Caplan, M., & Bennetto, L. (1988) *The Yale-New Haven social cognitive problem solving program for young adolescents*. New Haven, CT: Yale University Press.

Weissberg, R. P., Caplan, M., & Harwood, R. (1991). Promoting competent young people in competence-enhancing environments: A systems-based perspective on primary prevention. *Journal of Consulting and Clinical Psychology, 59*, 830–841.

Weissberg, R. P., Gesten, E. L., Rapkin, B. D., Cowen, E. L., Davidson, E., de Apodaca, R. F., & McKim, B. J. (1981). Evaluation of a social-problem-solving training program for suburban and inner-city third-grade children. *Journal of Consulting and Clinical Psychology, 49*, 251–261.

Wender, P. H. (1971). *Minimal brain dysfunction in children.* New York: Wiley.

Werry, J. S. (1968). Developmental hyperactivity. *Pediatric Clinics of North America, 19*, 9–16.

Werry, J. S., & Quay, H. C. (1971). The prevalence of behavior symptoms in younger elementary school children. *American Journal of Orthopsychiatry, 41*, 136–143.

Westman, J. C. (1990). *Handbook of learning disabilities: A multisystem approach.* Boston: Allyn and Bacon.

Whalen, C. K., & Henker, B. (1987). Cognitive–behavior therapy for hyperactive children: What do we know? In J. Loney (Ed.), *The young hyperactive child* (pp. 123–141). Birmingham, NY: Haworth.

Whitman, T. L., & Johnston, M. (1983). Teaching addition and substraction with regrouping to EMR children: A group self-instructional training program. *Behavior Therapy, 14*, 127–143.

Wilson, G. R. (1978). Cognitive–behavior therapy: Paradigm shift or passing phase? In J. P. Foreyt & D. P. Rathjen (Eds.), *Cognitive behavior therapy: Research and applications.* New York: Plenum Press.

Wirt, R. D., Lachar, D., Klinedinst, J. K., & Seat, P. D. (1984). *Multidimensional description of child personality: A manual for the Personality Inventory for Children* (rev. by D. Lachar). Los Angeles: Western Psychological Services.

Wong, B. Y. L., Harris, K., R., & Graham, S. (1991). Academic applications of cognitive-behavioral programs with learning-disabled students. In P. C. Kendall (Ed.), *Child and adolescent therapy: Cognitive–behavioral procedures* (pp. 245–275). New York: Guilford Press.

Wong, B. Y. L., & Jones, W. (1982). Increasing metacomprehension in learning-disabled and normally achieving students through self-questioning training. *Learning Disabilities Quarterly, 5*, 228–240.

Wright, J. C. (1973). *The KRISP: A technical report.* Unpublished manuscript.

Yeates, K. & Selman, R. L. (1989). Social competence in the schools: Toward an integrative developmental model for intervention. *Developmental Review, 9*, 64–100.

Ziegler, R., & Holden, L. (1988). Family therapy for learning-disabled and attention-deficit disordered children. *American Journal of Orthopsychiatry, 58*, 196–210.

Zivin, G. (Ed.). (1979). *The development of self-regulation through private speech.* New York: Wiley.

Index

CPSIA information can be obtained at www.ICGtesting.com
Printed in the USA
BVOW08*2336231215

430907BV00009B/293/P